T0187592

Forensic Mental Health Consulting in Family Law

Forensic Mental Health Professionals have entered the fray of child custody litigation in ways that could not have been predicted even a decade ago. Traditionally engaged as neutral court appointed evaluators or mediators, or as treatment providers for children, parents or families, FMHPs are assuming an array of consulting functions. Services span a wide range, including providing expert testimony on specific content areas; reviewing and critiquing colleague's work product; providing behind the scenes consultation to attorneys, and even helping attorneys manage difficult cases and clients. These more recent services raise questions about sound professional practice. *Forensic Mental Health Consulting in Family Law* tackles these thorny issues head on, and discusses questions of how consultants can work creatively and ethically to make a positive contribution in the challenging world of family law.

This book was originally published as a special issue of the *Journal of Child Custody*.

Robert L. Kaufman maintains a clinical and forensic practice in Oakland and San Rafael, California, USA. He is also a senior trial consultant with the San Francisco firm of Bonora D'Andrea, LLC.

S. Margaret Lee maintains a clinical and forensic practice in Mill Valley, California, USA devoted to divorcing families. Services include custody mediation and evaluation, training, co-parent counselling, expert testimony and consulting with attorneys.

Forensic Mental Health Consulting in Family Law

Part of the Problem or Part of the Solution?

Edited by
Robert L. Kaufman and S. Margaret Lee

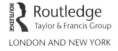

LONDON AND NEW YORK

First published 2012
by Routledge
2 Park Square, Milton Park, Abingdon, Oxon, OX14 4RN

Simultaneously published in the USA and Canada
by Routledge
711 Third Avenue, New York, NY 10017

Routledge is an imprint of the Taylor & Francis Group, an informa business

© 2012 Taylor & Francis

This book is a reproduction of the *Journal of Child Custody*, volume 8, issue 1-2. The Publisher requests to those authors who may be citing this book to state, also, the bibliographical details of the special issue on which the book was based.

All rights reserved. No part of this book may be reprinted or reproduced or utilised in any form or by any electronic, mechanical, or other means, now known or hereafter invented, including photocopying and recording, or in any information storage or retrieval system, without permission in writing from the publishers.

Trademark notice: Product or corporate names may be trademarks or registered trademarks, and are used only for identification and explanation without intent to infringe.

British Library Cataloguing in Publication Data
A catalogue record for this book is available from the British Library

ISBN13: 978-0-415-69793-4

Typeset in Baskerville
by Taylor & Francis Books

Disclaimer
The publisher would like to make readers aware that the chapters in this book are referred to as articles as they had been in the special issue. The publisher accepts responsibility for any inconsistencies that may have arisen in the course of preparing this volume for print.

Contents

Introduction

ROBERT L. KAUFMAN

Independent Practice, Oakland, California

S. MARGARET LEE

Independent Practice, Mill Valley, California

This special issue of the *Journal of Child Custody* is devoted to the exploration of emerging and evolving mental health consulting in family law. Certainly over the last five to ten years, it has become apparent that forensic mental health professionals (FMHPs) have been involving themselves in custody cases in ways that are moving afield from their historically traditional functions as court-appointed or private mediators, or neutral, court-appointed custody evaluators. During this period of time, many of us have seen changes in the family law landscape. Despite the fact that the courts are more and more crowded and under-resourced, litigation has become increasingly intense and contentious. The recent economic downturn has only amplified challenges for divorcing families.

At the same time, there has been a veritable explosion of wellgrounded, scientifically rooted research into some of the thorniest issues we see in custody cases. While definitive answers remain elusive, we now have deeper understanding of important issues such as alienation, and have better models and procedures for assessing abuse and domestic violence allegations and relocation cases, to name a few. At no time has it been more important for custody evaluators and others working in family law to keep abreast of the emerging literature.

It is heartening to see that at the same time that we are looking to broaden and refine our knowledge base and clinical skills, FMHPs are also engaged in examining how we go about our professional work. Within the past decade, we have seen a revision to the APA Guidelines for Child

Custody Evaluators in Family Law Proceedings (2009); Model Standards of Practice for Family and Divorce Mediation (AFCC 2000); Model Standards of Practice for Child Custody Evaluations (AFCC 2005); Guidelines for Parent Coordination (2005); and Guidelines for Brief Focused Assessment (AFCC 2009). And in progress is a revision to the *Specialty Guidelines for Forensic Psychology*. The AFCC has also convened a task force dedicated specifically to exploring practice issues of forensic mental health consulting in family law.

Thus, we have the exciting convergence of multiple forces, with professionals trying to work creatively, intelligently, and ethically in a demanding field where rewards can be high, but solutions are not always easy to come by. The FMHPs have jumped into the fray of custody litigation in ways that appear to be relatively new. Services to attorneys, parents, and the court have expanded and are not limited to "neutral" or court-appointed roles. We have more FMHPs working as consultants to attorneys on one side of a case, sometimes testifying, sometimes not. The functions can run the gamut. The FMHPs may be hired to provide expert testimony related to specific and discrete issues in the professional literature, or expand to a comprehensive review of a colleague's custody evaluation report. Attorneys have sought the assistance of FMHPs to manage difficult clients or to guide them through a custody evaluation. And, other professionals are teaming with attorneys to forge settlements via "hybrid" models.

There is no doubt in our minds that professionals can offer invaluable services that are innovative, respectful, and ethically responsible. But our expanding work is also raising questions as to what is ethical and what is helpful to the process of families and courts working to resolve complex and contentious matters in the best interest of children. Dialogues about consulting roles and services have become more frequent and at times heated. Ultimately we need to ask ourselves, are we part of the problem or part of the solution? That is, to what extent are we contributing to families being able to come to resolutions that address children's best interests versus how might these emerging roles and services be contributing to making an already difficult process more cumbersome, more contentious, and more expensive.

Along with journal editor Leslie Drozd, Ph.D., we felt it vital to put issues and questions on the table. This special issue of the *Journal of Child Custody* is an attempt to open up the discussion to the larger family law community. We are thrilled that a diverse group of seasoned and thoughtful professionals have contributed their ideas and experiences.

Robert Kaufman offers an historical perspective for consulting work in family law. Drawing on the evolution of both forensic psychology and trial consulting, he discusses how contributions from those fields can inform sound professional practice in family law consulting. He examines the complexities of the various relationships in FMHP family law consulting, and the challenges to the consultant to provide valued services to the retaining attorney and the parent/litigant, while respecting and addressing the best interests of the child. Guidelines for resolving possible conflicts are offered.

Jonathan Gould, David Martindale, Timothy Tippins, and Jeff Wittmann provide an in-depth discussion of the differences between consultants who are hired to provide testimony in court, and those who are retained to work behind the scenes in a confidential manner, assisting an attorney who is preparing for trial. The authors drill deeply into the complexities as well as the distinctions, noting that FMHPs can provide various services to attorneys within the general constructs of testifying versus non-testifying consulting. For them, an appreciation of the fundamental differences between the two roles will inform sound forensic consulting practice.

In their article, William G. Austin, Milfred D. Dale, H. D. Kirkpatrick, and James R. Flens address the consultation and work product review services that FMHPs provide in custody cases that are in litigation and where a child custody evaluation has been performed. These authors discuss both the challenges and responsibilities of the FMHP who is retained to review a colleague's custody evaluation for the purposes of the litigation. They further address issues that will soon become familiar to readers – the differences between consulting "roles" and "services," and the extent to which clear separations can be made between testifying and consulting services. The complex role of the Best Interests of the Child standard is also discussed.

S. Margaret Lee and Lorie S. Nachlis offer a "hybrid" model of consulting, aimed at assisting families in efforts to settle cases in ways that address children's needs and also circumvent litigation. They suggest that the retained consultant can serve different functions and offer various services depending on the specific needs of the family, and the specific point in the post-separation process. They believe that there are more options for families outside of court, and outline how FMHP consultant—attorneys teams can offer information and perspective often lost in intense litigation. They also discuss the professional issues inherent in working with such a model.

H. D. Kirkpatrick, William G. Austin, and James R. Flens offer new perspectives on both legal and psychological aspects of reviewing a colleague's child custody evaluation. In addition to addressing ethical and professional practice issues, the authors define ways in which review experts can assist the court. Beyond that, they also look at less overt or conscious psychological processes of both the reviewing expert and the evaluator whose work is being reviewed. The authors outline the responsibilities of the reviewing expert and suggest specific ways that evaluators can approach being reviewed. This article blends a conceptual framework with pragmatic practice guidelines.

We are especially pleased to have two commentary articles contributed by well-respected judicial officers. Hon. Mark Juhas has written a powerful and thoughtful piece about the day-to-day reality for a family court bench officer. His description of "what he sees," what he must deal with, and what he tries to accomplish each day is compelling reading. Judge Juhas offers his thoughts about how FMHPs can be helpful in the court process, and how they might impede the court's efforts. He discusses what he finds valuable in expert testimony, while always thinking of what serves the families who come to court in need of timely resolution to current conflicts.

Hon. Dianna Gould-Saltman brings a unique perspective to this issue. She is an experienced family law attorney who is now serving on the family law bench. In addition, she has a degree in psychology. As such, she offers experiences and views from these multiple points of view. Judge Gould-Saltman cogently elucidates what the various participants desire and antici-pate from family law proceedings, and cautions that not all judicial officers see their role in the same way. She goes on to discuss some of the expecta-tions on expert consultants, and offers keen insight into how bench officers may view testifying experts.

It is our sincere belief that the articles in this issue add to the on-going dialogue about FMHP consulting. There is no doubt we want to be "part of the solution." But, as any reader of this special issue will readily see, the issues are complex; thus the answers will also be complex. Thoughtful, respectful, and well informed discussion will advance the professional devel-opment of our field and advance our ultimate goal—to serve the interest of children and families at challenging junctures of life.

Forensic Mental Health Consulting in Family Law: Where Have We Come From? Where Are We Going?

ROBERT L. KAUFMAN

Independent Practice, Oakland, California

Forensic Mental Health Professionals (FMHPs) are venturing into a new and expanding form of consultation within the family law arena. They are more frequently being hired by attorneys on one side of a case to join the litigation team and perform a range of consulting functions that veer far afield from traditional FMHP roles as court appointed neutral evaluators and mediators. Though new and exciting opportunities are developing, FMHPs find themselves confronting dilemmas unique to these collaborations. The FMHPs must be answerable to the ethical standards of their profession, while accommodating the rules and needs of the legal world. Forensic psychologists have been involved in legal cases involving mental health issues for more than a hundred years. Trial consultants have also participated in trial preparation and research for more than thirty-five years. These professions have developed ethical and professional standards to guide their work. The FMHPs have much to gain from the efforts of these disciplines, as they endeavor to work responsibly with complex cases, highly charged issues, and multifaceted relationships.

Consider the following vignette: A skilled and experienced forensic psychologist and custody evaluator receives a call from a local attorney who is well respected in the local family law community. The psychologist has not worked with the attorney before, but is eager to establish a relationship with her and her firm, which often represent well-to-do parents and do not shy away from litigation.

The attorney needs help managing a difficult client who has recently begun going through a child custody evaluation. Despite the attorney's best efforts, the parent is constantly shooting himself in the foot. The parent is convinced that he is far smarter than the evaluator, believes that the evaluator has behaved unprofessionally, and is further convinced that the evaluator just does not like him. The parent argues directly with the evaluator and sends incendiary emails to his ex-wife. He is desperate to hang on to the time he has with his children, with whom he has been very actively involved.

The attorney believes sincerely that her client has been a good dad, and that while the dad may have some personal problems, his behavior primarily stems from his absolute panic about possibly losing time with his children. In her call to the psychologist, the attorney cries, "Help." If only a skilled forensic mental health professional could meet with the dad, help him understand what he is doing, and provide support and guidance for getting through the evaluation, he might have a shot at a reasonable outcome. The attorney needs help too, analyzing reams of documentation and developing a strategy for coping with the case she is facing.

A scenario such as this one is not as far fetched as one might think in the volatile and emotionally charged world of family law. The vignette represents some of the opportunities and fears of Forensic Mental Health Professionals (FMHPs) venturing into new territories in family law and custody consulting. On the one hand, this fictional consultant has been contacted by an attorney with whom he/she would very much like to develop an ongoing relationship. It would be awfully hard to turn down an invitation to work in a collaborative mode with a respected firm that could provide more work in the future. Plus, there is a lot of work to be done, at full consulting rate, and it could draw on the range of skills the FMHP has worked for years to hone—case analysis, knowledge of custody issues and evaluation procedures and clinical skills useful in dealing with difficult clients.

But on the other hand, has the attorney asked the consultant to do too much or to do something that would challenge the bounds of ethical behavior? What would be the impact of saying "no" to at least some of the attorney's requests? Is it acceptable practice to provide consultation to the attorney and also work with the parent? If so, what form should the work take? What kind of "guidance" is responsibly given to a parent who is going through a custody evaluation and could potentially be a witness in a custody proceeding? Is the work confidential? And, what if the dad turns out to be far more disturbed than the attorney believes? What would it mean to help a deeply troubled parent present well to a custody evaluator? Where does the best interest of the child standard fit into this picture?

As consultation services rapidly expand in family law cases, these are only some of the complex questions that as a profession, FMHPs need to be asking to ensure that we are delivering services that comport with sound and responsible professional practice. This is not a simple task. The FMHPs are being engaged by family law attorneys of one party to provide a variety of services, including but not limited to: reviewing and critiquing custody evaluations and mediation reports submitted to the court by neutral experts; assisting attorneys "behind the scenes" in various aspects of trial preparation; testifying in an educative manner on specific topics related to a case; offering rebuttal testimony; and even advising or "coaching" parents through custody proceedings. More traditionally used in neutral, court-appointed roles, FMHPs working in family law now find themselves on one side of a case, encountering the goals, wishes, desires, and, even at times, instructions of a particular attorney and a particular parent.

Some consulting roles are more established than others and have garnered more discussion in the professional literature. The FMHPs have been used with increased frequency to review or critique colleagues' work product and specifically custody evaluations at least since the mid 1990s. Such review work has been the subject of a number of articles addressing issues such as how FMHPs should approach such reviews, and what they add to the resolution of custody disputes (Stahl, 1996; Gould, Kirkpatrick, Austin, & Martindale, 2004). However, consulting roles for FMHPs in family law cases are still evolving, and FMHPs are becoming involved in custody matters in ways that could not have been predicted even in the last decade.

It is not hard to hypothesize why there is such an interest among forensic psychologists in developing these roles. Working within the legal framework can be an exciting and dynamic process, full of intellectual challenge. It also gets mental health professionals out of their individual practice milieus and more involved in a team approach to cases that can be emotionally draining and stressful to manage on one's own. Consulting work can also infuse diversity into a FMHP's practice, where there is always risk of burnout. And, with recent downturns in the economy, practitioners are seeking ways to distinguish themselves and diversify services they can offer.

Concurrently, many family law attorneys are utilizing FMHPs in ways that take better advantage of the range of the professional skills that a FMHP may have to offer. For example, skilled FMHPs can provide attorneys with knowledge of the ever-growing research on the many social and psychological factors inherent in the kinds of complex custody cases that often end up in contested hearings and trials. Or, given the increased emphasis on the science of custody evaluations, the FMHP may critique the thoroughness, methodology, and analysis of data collected for a custody evaluation. Newer roles seek to draw on the clinical skills of the FMHP, as family law attorneys seek their assistance in managing distraught, troubled or difficult clients, or to work actively and collaboratively to forge settlements and avoid lengthy and costly trials.

With these more recent functions, come increasingly complex relationships between psychologists and the individuals with whom they interact in family law cases. Traditionally, the legal arena is one predicated on an adversarial process, where argument based on evidence serves as the basis of determining the truth (Beck, Holtzworth-Munroe, D'Onofrio, Fee, & Hill, 2009). Working within the bounds of their own ethics, attorneys are expected to be zealous advocates for the clients. From this view, the FMHP is hired in the interest of furthering the case on behalf of the attorney's client, ostensibly with the goals of bolstering argument and ultimately winning the case. The attorney must advance, to the extent ethically permissible, the client's desired outcome. In family law, it may be an increase in custodial time, the ability to relocate with a child, the capacity to make child-rearing decisions unilaterally, or to oppose the other parent's request for such relief. At the same time that the consulting psychologist is there to be helpful to the retaining attorney whose client is a parent, the FMHP must also be cognizant of his/her own ethical responsibilities, including the obligation to work in the best interests of the child. As Shuman and Greenberg (2003) aptly noted, "the forensic expert is beholden to multiple masters. Integrating the demands of these masters is inherently complex" (p. 220). Thus, even though a family law consultant has entered into a formal contract with the attorney, these cases invariably involve multiple stakeholders, either directly or indirectly. And, not only must the consultant address demands and expectations from the attorney and the parent, he/she should always keep in mind who everyone is fighting about—the children.

As attorney-retained FMHPs become actively involved in more aspects of custody cases, they are also having increasing contact and interactions with the parents, who are the litigants in the case at hand. Given that FMHPs have joined the litigation "team" as consultants, they must consider the implications of their relationship with the parent-litigant, who invariably brings an impassioned investment in the outcome of the case. This in turn, can create strong pulls on the FMHP to join in the advocacy process. By way of example, consider the dilemma for the consultant who is brought in to support a parent's petition to relocate with a child. What if after immersing him/herself in the case, the consultant comes to believe that such a move would create undue stress or detriment to the child? What does the consultant do with his/her opinions? And, while rarely talked about, it is also the parent who is funding the attorney's work, which now includes the consultant. Thus, with the introduction of direct contact with the parent, the "multiple masters" have increased in numbers.

As consultants become more prevalent in custody litigation, and as FMHP-attorney collaborations expand in new directions, it seems important and worthwhile to pause and consider thoughtfully just what it is we are doing. What are the parameters of our role as consultants and the various services provided? What are the ethical issues of professional practice when a consultant works with within the legal arena but is bound by the ethics of professional mental health practice? How can FMHP consultants observe their own professional standards when working collaboratively with attorneys whose professional standards may differ from those of the consultant?

This article suggests that there is much to be learned from an historical view of the interface of mental health professionals and the legal system as we consider the ethical and professional complexities of consulting relationships. To that end, it is suggested that we can look to two vital sources—the evolution of forensic psychology and trial consulting—to guide our thinking. While FMHP consultation is a relatively new phenomenon in family law matters, psychologist mental health professionals have provided testimony in court proceedings for more than a century. For the majority of that time, FMHPs, and in particular forensic psychologists, have been engaged in expert testimony, assisting the trier of fact to understand mental health issues of individuals in cases before the court. In these roles, FMHPs have tried to bring to the legal venue the strengths of a scientific approach to understanding people along with clinical acumen. At the same time, forensic psychologists have learned that they must be mindful of the "rules" of a profession that is not their own. The competent and responsible FMHP must know the legal standards, precedents, and rulings that apply in the specific area in which they practice, as their work must be oriented to the psycho-legal questions at hand. As they have gained a firmer footing in the courtroom, forensic psychologists have worked hard to address issues of professional practice and ethics (Weissman & DeBow, 2003).

For at least the past 35 years, social scientists of various disciplines have also provided consultation in other aspects of trial proceedings. In contrast to forensic mental health consulting, trial consultation has received far more attention and scrutiny in the professional literature in terms of the direct application of social science to the legal process (Kovera, Dickinson, & Cutler, 2003). Initially growing out of a specific set of legal cases, and spurred on by a sense of social activism, trial consultants today assist attorneys in remarkably diverse ways and in an enormously varied range of cases, large and small. For example, they assist attorneys with pre- and post-trial research, case strategy, venue analysis, jury selection, and witness preparation. As such, trial consultants are hired to join litigation teams that are sometimes composed of attorneys from multiple law firms, even representing multiple clients. Many trial consultants are asked to work not only with the attorneys, but also directly with litigants and participants in the trial. Thus, they too are involved in complex relationships where professional standards and responsibility must be woven into the intense team drive to win the case (Lieberman & Sales, 2007). Trial consultants, some of whom are FMHPs, have also sought to define themselves professionally and to develop a set of standards and ethics to guide their work. This article will draw on these sources to understand the complexities of the relationships implied in the emerging roles for consulting FMHPs in family law, as they endeavor to serve the needs of the retaining attorney, the parent-litigant, the court's goal to find the truth, and last, but certainly not least, the best interests of the child.

This article does not presume to prescribe definitive answers to these difficult questions; it is intended to highlight what we know from these two areas of practice to inform discourse from which solutions can emerge. Given the relative wealth of discussion in the literature of models for conducting reviews of colleagues' work products, and specifically child custody evaluations, this article will turn most of its attention to the other emerging consulting roles in family law.

DEFINING THE INTERSECTION OF PSYCHOLOGY AND LAW

While not all FMHPs are psychologists, the intersection of the mental health and legal professions is best described in the literature of forensic psychology. There are several accessible definitions of forensic psychology. "Specialty Guidelines for Forensic Psychology" were originally drafted and approved by the American Psychology-Law Society, Division 41 of the American Psychological Association (APA) and the American Board of Forensic Psychology in 1991 (Committee on Ethical Guidelines for Forensic Psychologists, 1991) and are currently in the process of revision. The most recent revision (August 2010) defines forensic psychology as "all professional practice by any psychologist working within any subdiscipline of psychology (e.g., clinical, developmental, social, cognitive) when applying the scientific, technical, or specialized knowledge of psychology to the law to assist in addressing legal, contractual, and administrative matters." It seems important to emphasize that the *Specialty Guidelines* are not intended to apply to an individual's typical area of practice or expertise, but to "the service provided in the case at hand" (Revision p. 3).

Furthermore, professional practice is considered to be forensic not just because it takes place in the courtroom or judicial procedure per se, but because it addresses specific psycho-legal questions or issues. Goldstein (2003, p. 4) suggests that forensic psychology "involves the application of psychological research, theory, practice and traditional and specialized methodology (e.g., interviewing, psychological testing, forensic assessment, and forensically relevant instruments) to provide information relevant to a legal question." As such, FMHPs provide "products" (such as reports and testimony) to "consumers" (e.g., judges, attorneys) that contain information to aid in legal decision-making. The *Specialty Guidelines* thereby suggest that forensic psychologists should be, in a sense, responsive to *both* the profession that credentials them, as well as the profession that establishes the rules of applicability.

Among the examples of forensic services typically rendered by FMHPs noted in the *Specialty Guidelines* is "serving as a trial consultant or otherwise offering expertise to attorneys, the courts, or others" (Revision, p. 3). Section 1.04 specifically outlines that forensic practice may include not only examination and assessment of an individual's functioning, but also consultation regarding the "practical implications of relevant research, examination findings, and the opinions of other psycho-legal experts" (Revision, p. 3). Thus, consultants in the Family Law arena should know that their work not only has historical precedence, but can be considered to fall under the umbrella of at least one set of guiding principles for ethical professional practice. Though the *Specialty Guidelines* remain aspirational, they provide important considerations of relevant and sometimes controversial matters of forensic mental health consulting in Family Law, including representation of competencies, knowledge of the legal system, multiple relationships, privacy, confidentiality, and privilege.

EARLY INVOLVEMENT OF PSYCHOLOGISTS IN LEGAL PROCEEDINGS

How psychologists made their way into the courtroom is not only an interesting story, but shows that the roots of professional forensic practice can be found in the early stages of the profession.

The early direct or "real world" application of psychology and the law can be traced to the writings of Hugo Münsterberg (1906, 1908, 1909, 1914) at the beginning of the 20th century. By that time, many areas of science had been recognized as having application in the courtroom, starting with microscopy and toxicology. However, psychology, the relatively young but rapidly growing and arguably the leading American field of social science, had been excluded. In 1908, Münsterberg, a Harvard psychologist, thrust himself in the middle of debates as to whether psychology had any applicability in legal matters by commenting on the validity of the confession given by an accused murderer who had mental limitations. Though unsuccessful in getting the court to reconsider its actions in the specific case, Münsterberg went on to publish *On the Witness Stand* (1908), an edited collection of eight popular articles written about legal psychology. Among the topics considered by Münsterberg were the memories of witnesses, hypnosis and crime, and the reliability and veracity of confessions. While Münsterberg's commentaries might seem crude or hyperbolic by today's standards, his opinions opened up many areas of exploration within the legal arena pertinent to the science of psychology, for example pushing the issue that the accuracy of a witness' testimony could be influenced by his/her state of mind and/or cognitive capacities.

Unfortunately, Münsterberg's (1908) articles were more popular than scientific, lacking references and not offering adequate scientific foundation to gain acknowledgement, much less admissibility in the courtroom. Münsterberg also took the legal profession to task for its own "unscientific" approach. Münsterberg's writings were the brunt of a scathing and satirical attack by John H. Wigmore, the Dean of Northwestern Law School (1913), which no doubt delayed the acceptance of psychology by the legal profession at least 20 years (Goldstein, 2003, p. 7).

Also, at the beginning of the 20th century, William Marston (Marston, 1917), a student of Münsterberg's at Harvard, found correspondence between an individual's blood pressure and the truthfulness of his/her statements. Marston's studies formed the basis of the polygraph, but perhaps just as important, he was brought in as a defense expert in the trial of James Frye in 1922. Marston was asked to apply his "deception" test to a recanted confession by the defendant. The argument over the admissibility of Marston's testimony took on meaning beyond the case itself. In 1923, the Court of Appeals of the District of Columbia submitted a written decision that established the standard for admissibility of scientific evidence in federal court. What is known in California and elsewhere as the Kelly-Frye standard was stated in its original form in *Frye v. United States* (1923) 293 F.1013. The Kelly-Frye standard mandates that new scientific evidence must be relevant to the case and generally accepted within the relevant portions of the scientific community. It excludes from evidence any test results from scientifically unproven methods. This "general-acceptance" standard is still in place in some states (Ogloff & Finkelman, 1999).

As scientific evidence in the courtroom advanced, the Supreme Court recognized that a broader test for admissibility of scientific evidence was required to allow federal judges to perform their gate-keeping function in light of the Federal Rules of Evidence which had been enacted after *Frye*. In *Daubert v. Merrell Dow Pharmaceuticals, Inc.* (1993), the Supreme Court directed federal judges to assess the admissibility of expert evidence based not just on general acceptance in the scientific community, but also on whether a determination could be made as to whether the evidence could be tested and shown to be reliable. Expert evidence now had to be grounded specifically in scientific methodology. As the ruling explained, it could no longer be assumed that evidence was accurate and scientific simply because it was introduced by an expert in a field and generally accepted by their peers. Witnesses had to explain the bases of their opinions, and establish that these bases were rooted in scientific inquiry and methodology (Goodman-Delahunty, 1997; Kelly & Ramsey, 2007).

In the several decades following the *Frye* decision, psychological testimony in the courtroom was limited to testimony or consultation in a number of high profile criminal cases, with more significant growth occurring after World War II. Marston, for example, was called to provide consultation in the Lindbergh baby kidnapping case in 1932. And, also in that matter, New York City psychiatrist Dr. Dudley Shoenfeld, filed a report with the New York City Police Department containing a psychological profile of the kidnapper after studying the ransom notes that were sent to the family. Interestingly, this profile turned out to be remarkably accurate.

The application of psychological research to court decisions took a significant leap in the 1954 U.S. Supreme Court decision in *Brown v. Board of Education*. The decision declared that the discriminatory nature of racial segregation . . . "violates the 14th amendment to the U.S. Constitution, which guarantees all citizens equal protection of the laws." At trial in *Brown*'s consolidated case *Briggs v. Elliott*, the National Association for the Advancement of Colored People (NAACP) presented testimony by psychologist Kenneth B. Clark of the City College of New York. During the 1940s, Clark and his wife designed a test utilizing dolls of different skin color, and drawing tasks to study the psychological effects of segregation on black children. The NAACP legal team argued that Clark's findings demonstrated the detrimental effect of segregation on the psychological development of African-American children. The Supreme Court specifically cited Clark's 1950 paper in the *Brown* decision, using directly mental health and social science research to inform legal decision-making (Beggs, 1995).

As psychological research and practice were growing and developing, its acceptance in court was still slow to emerge. In 1962, the U.S. District Court for the Washington D.C. Circuit held that non-medical mental health professionals, including psychologists, were qualified to offer expert opinions in court regarding mental disorders at the time a crime was committed (*Jenkins v. United States* 1962). Heretofore, this was the exclusive domain of medical professionals. In *Jenkins*, the court stated that some psychologists are qualified to render opinions about mental disorders, provided they were sufficiently competent to do so. This was a matter of the psychologist's experience, expertise and the probative value of his/her opinions.

The foundation for forensic mental health consulting was established in *Ake v. Oklahoma* (1985). In this criminal case, the U.S. Supreme Court affirmed that a mental health expert or consultant could be a viable member of a defense or prosecution team. In addition to conducting forensic mental health evaluations of defendants for an attorney on one side of the case, the forensic psychology expert could also provide an analysis of relevant case themes, feedback on the strengths and weaknesses of the opposing side's case themes and review the opposing expert's assessments (Drogin, 2007). Thus, defense attorneys could obtain consulting assistance that went beyond simply obtaining rebuttal forensic mental health assessments.

ETHICAL GUIDELINES FOR FORENSIC PSYCHOLOGISTS

A younger field than either law or medicine, the American Psychological Association (APA) first instituted a code of ethical and professional conduct in 1953 (APA, 1953 and 1959).

As noted, it was not until the 1962 U.S. Supreme Court decision in *Jenkins v. United States* that courts recognized that psychologists with specific training and expertise could offer testimony in court regarding mental disease or illness. As psychologists were increasingly involved in legal cases, reference to forensic practice also made its way into the APA ethics code revisions. The APA 1992 revision included a separate section on forensic activities, thus affirming it as a unique domain of practice in psychology (Lipsitt, 2007). While references to forensic activities remained in the APA ethics code, a far more detailed discussion of professional practice and ethical issues was provided in the *Specialty Guidelines for Forensic Psychologists* in 1991. Nonetheless, APA did not recognize forensic psychology as a specialty area of practice until 2002.

The practice of forensic psychology involves professionals who are ethically responsible to the tenets of their discipline, but who also must accommodate the rules of another (Lipsitt, 2007). Both the APA ethics code and the *Specialty Guidelines* recognize the potential for conflicts between ethics and the law. This is acknowledged and discussed, for example in APA Ethics Code section 1.02 (Conflicts Between Ethics and Law, Regulations, or Other Governing Legal Authority) as well as other sections that address issues of confidentiality and privacy (Section 4.01), Multiple Relationships (Section 3.05), and Conflict of Interest (Section 3.06).

The *Specialty Guidelines* address a range of potentially conflict-laden issues for the forensic consultant, from the responsibility to clarify the consulting agreement at the onset, to the conflicts between therapeutic and forensic roles. It seems important to remember that the *Specialty Guidelines* do not offer absolutes, but rather some guidance to navigate responsibly almost inevitable conundrums and complexities when psychologists work in the legal arena. Though it may appear to be obvious on the surface, it bears repeating that fundamental abiding principles spelled out in the *Specialty Guidelines* can often inform ethical practice:

- Integrity: "Forensic practitioners seek to promote accuracy, honesty, and truthfulness in the science, teaching, and practice of forensic psychology and they strive to resist partisan pressures to provide services in any ways that might tend to be misleading or inaccurate" (3.01).
- Impartiality and Fairness: "Forensic practitioners recognize the adversarial nature of the legal system and strive to treat all participants and weigh all data, opinions, and rival hypotheses objectively" (3.02).
- Avoiding Conflicts of Interest: "Forensic practitioners refrain from taking on a professional role when personal, scientific, professional, legal, financial, or other interest or relationships could reasonably be expected to impair their objectivity, competence, or effectiveness, or expose other with whom a professional relationship exists to harm" (3.03).

HISTORY OF TRIAL CONSULTING

The history of trial consulting and specifically the application of social science to jury selection can be traced to the work of academic researchers in the 1971–1972 criminal trials of the Harrisburg Seven. In this case, a group of anti-war activists, including Father Philip Berrigan, were accused of several crimes including conspiring to destroy draft board records and kidnap Henry Kissinger, then a presidential advisor. Though the alleged crimes were said to have occurred in various other cities, federal prosecutors selected Harrisburg, Pennsylvania as the site for the trial, given their understanding that it was a politically conservative area. The defense recruited a team of social scientists headed by Jay Schulman of Columbia University to survey Harrisburg residents, both on the phone and face to face. Based on this research, the consultants fashioned profiles of jurors who were likely to be biased against the defense case, an approach that is still fundamental to jury selection. The defense trial team relied on this initial jury consulting method to choose the jury. In this politically conservative venue, and despite the fact that the government had spent more than $2 million on the prosecution of the case, the jury was deadlocked with 10 jurors favoring acquittal and 2 jurors favoring conviction. No retrial took place (Lieberman & Sales, 2007; Strier, 1999; Kairys, 2008).

Schulman then applied the jury selection consulting methodology to other cases, including the Wounded Knee trials. The techniques developed were then applied to numerous other political criminal cases. Since that time, trial consulting has also garnered considerable public attention, and not inconsiderable controversy, in many high-profile cases such as the trials of OJ Simpson, the Menendez brothers, Rodney King, Kobe Bryant, Martha Stewart, Michael Jackson, and Scott Peterson.

While trial consulting has been most visible to the public in highly publicized criminal cases, where the consulting world has really boomed is in civil litigation (Lieberman & Sales, 2007). The field saw rapid growth through the 1980s, as trial consultants became involved in large, highly publicized and diverse civil matters, such as class action lawsuits against tobacco companies and the McDonald's coffee-spill case. In the world of big money, high-stakes litigation, trial consultants virtually became the norm, rather than the exception.

WHO ARE TRIAL CONSULTANTS?

Trial consultants work in various phases of litigation, engaging contractually with an attorney or law firm to become part of the litigation team. Among the services that trial consultants provide in litigation that may be of interest to FMHPs in family law include:

- Case analysis and strategy: Reviewing case materials to analyze compelling themes; evaluating strengths and weaknesses of the case from both sides; developing narratives and arguments for trial presentation.
- Witness preparation: This may include working directly with lay and/or expert witnesses, and can include discussion, review of prior testimony through recordings and/or transcripts, or mock testimony.
- Presentation strategy: This may include discussion with attorneys regarding the relative strength of evidence to be presented at trial, as well as the means of presentation. There may be development of presentation tools, such as graphic displays of evidence or argument.
- Examination strategy: Reviewing with attorneys how they will conduct both direct and cross examination of lay and expert witnesses. This could include general discussions, or assistance crafting specific examination questions.

Other trial consulting roles, less directly applicable to family law consulting, include offering direct input and assistance with jury selection, including voir dire strategy; conducting focus groups and mock trials to understand attitudes and opinions about a specific case or relevant case themes; providing consultation on opening and closing statements; conducting community attitude surveys and change of venue surveys. Trial consultants may also appear as expert witnesses, such as in change of venue research.

It is important to keep in mind that trial consultants are a heterogeneous group of professionals that includes FMHPs of different disciplines, social scientists, academics, attorneys, and communications experts. There are no specific educational requirements for becoming a trial consultant and there is no certification that must be obtained. While family law mental health consultants may also be of different disciplines (e.g., psychologists, social workers), they are most typically individuals who are licensed to practice in their profession, with their professional activities overseen by licensing or credentialing boards. Thus, professional and ethical standards are in place, though the direct applicability of those standards to consulting work remains less than crystal clear. Still, how trial consultants have addressed professional standards issues may still be instructive.

PROFESSIONAL DEVELOPMENT OF TRIAL CONSULTING

In 1982, a group of consultants gathered to form a professional organization to address the needs and interests of litigation consultants. Initially known as the Association of Trial Behavior Consultants, the organization originally had twenty-four members. In 1985, the name of the group changed to its present form, the American Society of Trial Consultants (ASTC), and there are currently roughly five hundred members. In the early years of ASTC, a number of members pushed to develop professional standards, feeling that it would both legitimize the emerging profession, and insulate consultants to some degree from possible lawsuits by disgruntled clients (A. Sheldon,

	Timeline of key events in evolution of forensic psychology and trial consulting
1908	H. Munsterberg, Harvard psychologist, publishes *On the Witness Stand*, which includes eight essays on legal psychology
1909	Munsterberg's essays are challenged by J. Wigmore, Dean of Northwestern Law School
1922	W. Marston, a developer of the "deception" test, appears as defense witness in *Frye v. United States*
1923	*Frye* decision on admissibility of scientific evidence: relevant to the case and generally accepted within the relevant portions of the scientific community
1932	Lindbergh baby case: Marston testifies; first psychological profiling in a criminal case
1952	APA's first code of ethics and professional practice. No mention of forensic work
1954	*Brown v. Board of Education:* Supreme Court use of mental health testing and research to inform legal decision-making
1962	*Jenkins v. US:* Psychologists are qualified to render opinions about mental disorders, provided they were sufficiently competent to do so
1971	Social scientist research and consultants used in defense cases against anti-war activists.
1982	Formation of Association of Trial Behavior Consultants, which became American Society of Trial Consultants
1985	*Ake v. Oklahoma* Mental health expert or consultant could be part of litigation team and not just an evaluator of individuals
1991	*Specialty Guidelines for Forensic Psychologists* American Psychology-Law Society and Division 41 of APA
1992	APA Code of ethics and professional practice includes specific section on forensic psychology
1993	*Daubert v. Merrell Dow Pharmaceuticals, Inc.* Expert evidence now had to be grounded specifically in scientific methodology (can be tested and shown to be reliable
2003	*In re: Cendant Corporation:* upheld attorney work product protections for trial consultants, including working with witnesses.
2008	Most recent revision of the Professional Code of ASTC

FIGURE 1 Historical timeline of forensic psychology and trial consulting.

personal communication, September 21, 2010). By virtue of education, professional affiliation and experience, ASTC's membership was diverse. And, with practitioners engaging in such a range of services, it was initially impossible to get consensus on a unified set of practice and ethical guidelines.

The committee working on developing guidelines first started with a survey of membership to determine interests and attitudes. It was decided not to tackle the guidelines in a comprehensive manner, but rather to see in what specific practice areas members could agree to a set of standards. Thus, ASTC first adopted guidelines for venue survey research. In all, there are five separate areas, the other four being: Witness Preparation, Small Group Research, Jury Selection, and Post Trial Juror Interviews.

The most recent revision of the *Professional Code of ASTC* was in 2008. As with the *Specialty Guidelines for Forensic Psychology*, the code is primarily aspirational in nature. "The Practice Guidelines are informative only and are not meant to be comprehensive, exclusive or to supplant the professional judgment of a consultant" (p. 1). ASTC has, however, set up a grievance procedure and has fielded a relatively small number of complaints. As there is no specific credential for trial consulting, and as ASTC is a professional organization and not an oversight board, they have few remedies for violations of the professional code.

Even so, some specific aspects of the *Professional Code of ASTC* may be informative for FMHPs working in family law. As with the *Guidelines for Forensic Psychology*, the code does not always answer particular ethical or professional dilemmas, but it can raise the right questions and guide thinking through issues at hand. Figure 1 summarizes key dates in the history of forensic psychology and trial consulting.

ATTORNEY-CONSULTANT RELATIONSHIP

There can be strong pulls on the FMHP consultant to please the retaining attorney. Pulls, both conscious and unconscious, can go beyond the desire to deliver competent, insightful and timely services. As part of the "litigation team," the FMHP can easily be drawn into the attorney's advocacy perspective, including the attorney's responsibility to work diligently on behalf of his/her client (Greenberg & Shuman, 2007). While attorneys no doubt know that licensed mental health professionals must be responsive to professional codes of ethics, and are answerable to licensing boards, they cannot be expected to appreciate thornier ethical dilemmas. Attorneys do not always understand the limits of what services psychologist consultants can offer and what roles they can responsibly assume. Both the *Specialty Guidelines for Forensic Psychology* and the *Professional Code of ASTC* emphasize the importance of establishing a clear contract and setting expectations between the retaining party and the consultant. With the expansion of litigation consultation in so many forms, it seems imperative that the attorney and consultant enter into a written contract that spells out expectations. The *Specialty Guidelines* make distinctions between the relationship established with the retaining party and the relationships with "those with whom they interact (e.g., examinees, collateral contacts, research participants, students)" (Section 6). Implied in the section called Responsibilities to Retaining Parties is that a contract between the retaining party (usually the attorney) and the consultant is necessary, and that at the time the contract is discussed, the FMHPs "seek to clarify the nature of the relationship and the services to be provided including the role of the forensic practitioner...; which person or entity is the client; the probable uses of the services provided or information obtained; and any limitations to privacy, confidentiality, or privilege" (Section 6.01). Presumably, this would include whether the FMHP is likely to be a consultant "behind the scenes" or possibly a testifying expert. This, of course, has implications for whether the work will be protected by attorney work product.

The *Professional Code of ASTC* suggests that close scrutiny needs to be paid to precisely who the retaining party is. The trial consultant is most commonly retained directly by an attorney or law firm and becomes part of the litigation team. However, there may be times when retention comes from the client whom the attorney is representing, or even from an insurance company who is contractually financing the litigation. The question of who is the client is an important one. As the *Professional Code* spells out, "the trial consultant who is retained by the attorney: (1) works under the direction and supervision of the attorney; (2) cooperates with the attorney to assure all consultant-attorney communication is subject, to the extent provided under the law, to attorney/client privilege and work-product doctrine" (Page 4). When the contract is made with the litigant, the work "probably is not subject to legal protection from discloser under any attorney/client privilege, work-product, or other doctrine" (Page 4).

It is this author's experience that most family law consultants understand that they need to work with a written contract, and that the contract should be with the attorney who represents the party or parent. However, there are no standards for contracts and the matter of who provides payment for services and at what time is less clear. Even some experienced attorneys prefer that their clients (the parent-litigant) pay consultants directly. The attorney may not want to incur the liability for the consultant directly, especially if they are having trouble collecting fees from the parent/litigant. This can be a dangerous practice on several fronts, as it surely jeopardizes the objectivity of the consultant, who may well feel that payment for services is somehow dependent on how their opinions are received by the parent. Sound forensic practice includes contracting directly with the attorney for a retainer at the onset of the consultation agreement and obtaining additional monies when those retainers are depleted.

In light of these considerations, FMHP consultants would be well advised to:

- Always work from a written contract that spells out the terms of the consulting agreement. The agreement should include:
  - The scope and nature of anticipated work;
  - The intention that information gathered and opinions rendered will remain confidential and held under privilege to the extent provided by law;
  - Any potential limits to confidentiality that can be anticipated at the onset of the agreement, including but not limited to the possibility that the consultant will be a testifying expert;
  - Responsibilities of the retaining party and the consultant under the contract;
  - Explicit fee agreement; and
  - How the consultation agreement can be terminated by either party.
- Establish the contract should be between the consultant and the retaining attorney;
- Work with a retainer system and avoid accepting contingent fees; and
- Accept payments directly by the attorney and not by the litigating or other third party.

The consulting agreement sets the framework and the tone for attorney-consultant relationship. Fortunately, the principles of science can anchor the FMHP consultant as he or she navigates the waters between advocacy and neutrality. The objectivity of the scientific process underlies admissibility under *Daubert*, including the mandate to weigh the relative merits of rival hypotheses, and discusses the basis for the opinions rendered. These criteria are echoed in several sections of the *Specialty Guidelines* in phrases such as "truthfulness in science," "goals of accuracy, objectivity, fairness and independence." Thus, the competent and respected FMHP consultant will best serve the retaining attorney via the consultant's independent ability to view the strengths and weaknesses of the case. This represents the consultant's sound understanding of the adversarial process and their responsibilities within it. (Shuman & Greenberg, 2003) So, rather than shying away from exploring fully the relative merits of the opposing case, consultants should see this as a responsible part of the consulting practice. It is hoped that FMHP consultants who are known for their objectivity and independence will earn a sound reputation in the legal community. In fact, a consultant's ability to point out the weaknesses in a case can be an invaluable asset in an attorney's responsibility to help the parent-litigant come to agreements or settlements that are more realistic than their expectations.

CONSULTANT-PARENT RELATIONSHIP

Increasingly, FMHP consultants are having direct contact and interactions with the retaining attorney's client—the parent. Again, roles may be diverse. As outlined by Hobbs-Minor and Sullivan (2008), there is much to be gained by affording parents sound and responsible consultation in the context of the attorney-client relationship. Therapeutic support, education about divorce-related issues including children's developmental needs, and realistic views of custody proceedings can all contribute to better outcomes for families. Conceived in part as an expanded conflict resolution role, there can be direct benefits to the parents, the parent's attorney, and indirectly to children and even other family members. However, consultants and parents also enter into relationships that are complex and demand that the FMHP exercise particular care, caution, and expertise. As those authors also point out, role boundaries and ethical practice issues have not been well explored in the literature.

The distinctions between therapeutic and forensic roles have been well discussed in the forensic psychology literature (e.g., Heilbrun, 2001; Greenberg & Shuman, 1997, 2007). Those discussions, which need not be repeated here, have focused primarily on forensic assessment of individuals versus therapeutic assessment and treatment. Many of the principles of forensic assessment surely apply to FMHP consulting. For example, the consultation work is performed in the context of a legal action and must address relevant psycho-legal questions; the consultant should remain neutral, at least quasi-objective and explore all facets of the case; the work involves a multi-client system.

In expanded consulting roles involving parents, distinctions between forensic and therapeutic roles become less clear. Hobbs-Minor and Sullivan (2008) note that in some roles, direct and substantive contact with the parent is an essential part of the process that is deemed helpful:

> The mental health consultant: (1) provides support to the parent and to the attorney in obtaining the most recent information and expertise that can assist with the specifics needed on the case; (2) teaches the parent new skills to move towards resolution of custody issues; (3) collaborates with the attorney and the parent as a team throughout the mediation and/or family court process; (4) remains under the confidentiality of the attorney-client privileged relationship; and (5) serves as a parenting plan advisor (Hobbs-Minor, 1998).

As these authors note, the skilled FMHP consultant can bring a beneficial perspective to the parent as they try to resolve post-divorce custody disputes. They can provide educational information; help manage parents' anxieties and fears; offer direct feedback to parents about their views and perspectives; assist parents to remain child-focused; and offer psychological structuring to emotionally vulnerable parents (Hobbs-Minor & Sullivan 2008).

In addition, some consultants are hired to offer parents advice on how to manage their participation in a custody evaluation.

These more recent family law consulting roles raise several questions. Among them is to the extent to which consultant-parent contact is confidential and protected by attorney work-product privilege. The Supreme Court first recognized this privilege in 1947 in *Hickman v. Taylor*, 329 U.S. 495, 510–11 (1947). In that decision, the Court held that an attorney must "work with a certain degree of privacy, free from unnecessary intrusion by opposing parties and their counsel" and be free to "assemble information, sift what he considers to be the relevant from the irrelevant facts, prepare his legal theories and plan his strategy without undue and needless interference." The context of attorney work-product protection in current or anticipated litigation extends to experts and consultants hired by attorneys, so long as the FMHP has not been designated as a testifying expert.

While there is good reason for consultants to have confidence in the protection of attorney work-product, the trial consulting literature suggests that some caveats and cautions should be exercised (Perrott & Wolfe, 2010). This issue has been explored in some depth in the trial consulting literature, where attorneys and consultants are highly invested in keeping pre-trial research, preparation and jury selection strategy private and confidential. The case most often referred to is *In re: Cendant Corpor.* (2003) which generally upheld protections established in *Hickman v. Taylor* as applied to trial consultant's work. (Interestingly, the consultant who provided witness preparation in the Cendant matter was Dr. Phillip McGraw, better known as "Dr. Phil.") *In re: Cendant* was argued and appealed, with the final ruling made by the U.S. Court of Appeals for the Third District. In most jurisdictions, the ability of an attorney to discover a consultant's work has not been fully resolved (ASTC Professional Code p. 34). That is to say, it appears that the *Cendant* decision protects the content of the consultant's work with witnesses under attorney work-product, but not necessarily the fact that the consultant was used. And, even this cannot be guaranteed. Thus, it is possible that a parent who has worked with a mental health consulting expert might have to acknowledge that they worked with a consultant, and who the consultant was, though it is unclear as to whether they would have to testify as to the exact content of meetings and discussions with the FMHP consultant. On the surface, this might not seem problematic. However, even the mere acknowledgment that a parent has worked with a consultant can be viewed negatively by a custody evaluator or can be cannon fodder for an aggressive attorney on the other side. Custody evaluators may feel uncomfortable knowing that there is someone with whom the parent is discussing the evaluation process, and may not trust that the parent is really being themselves in interviews and observations. And, opposing counsel may cast doubt on the credibility of a parent who has worked with a consultant, even if the consultant has acted in very responsible ways. This certainly should signal family law mental health consultants that they must be very careful in terms of how they support and advise the parents with whom they meet.

Parent-Consultant Meetings—Witness Preparation?

While not all parents whose attorneys have engaged a consulting FMHP are on track for a full custody trial, it should be acknowledged that most parents testify in court or provide sworn declarations at custody proceedings. Even if the consultant is not asked to meet with the parent specifically to discuss his/her testimony in court, a consultant's input may also affect parents' participation in custody evaluations, statements in hearings or settlement conferences and family court mediation. Apart from issues of confidentiality noted previously, what are some of the ethical considerations of working with parents who are going through custody proceedings?

The trial consulting literature can again afford some perspective here. Of the many diverse services that trial consultants have provided, working with witnesses in preparation for trial is the most controversial. It is performed by consultants of various disciplines, and can range in scope from offering coaching about dress, demeanor, and presentation style, to engaging in very detailed mock direct and cross-examinations. While much of this may not appear to pertain directly to the custody consultant working with a parent in litigation, some principles are surprisingly relevant.

Trial consultants are often brought in on cases where there are high personal and financial stakes, and where pressures for witnesses to "perform" well in court are enormous. It is very easy for the trial consultant to join in the pressure-cooker atmosphere that is the norm in trial preparation. In terms of working with witnesses, attorneys are primarily guided by the American Bar Association's Model Rules of Professional Conduct (1983) which prohibits attorneys from falsifying evidence or assisting witnesses to testify untruthfully. Interestingly, until ASTC developed professional standards, there were no parallel guidelines for consultants who were part of the attorney team. Trial consulting professional standards attempt to address the complex dynamics and responsibilities inherent in working with potential witnesses. Some of the questions the standards try to address include: who should be doing witness preparation; the need for informed consent; are there any guidelines for determining ethical versus unethical consultation. Several components of the ASTC standards seem directly relevant to the hybrid roles FMHPs are assuming that include supporting or collaborating with parents who are involved in custody proceedings:

- Trial consultants shall advocate that a witness tell the truth;
- Trial consultants shall provide witness preparation services within the boundaries of their competence based on education, training, or other appropriate professional experience;

- Trial consultants shall discuss with the client limitations on confidentiality in the provision of witness preparation services including but not limited to discovery requests; and
- Trial consultants do not script specific answers or censor appropriate and relevant answers based solely on the expected harmful effect on case outcome.

The FMHP consultant who finds him/herself working directly with parents has many goals that seem reasonable and even admirable. Is it not reasonable to help a parent express themselves more effectively to a custody evaluator or even on the witness stand? Is it not helpful to assist the parent to see multiple sides of a complex situation and wade through the pros and cons of various custody schedules they might propose to an evaluator? Should a parent not be well versed in the issues relevant to petitions to relocate with a child and be able to address these issues in an evaluation or court hearing?

In developing guidelines for professional practice, ASTC struggled with the ethics of advising and preparing witnesses, especially making distinctions between providing information, feedback and guidance, versus unethical approaches such as scripting, shaping, and instructing witnesses. Instructive in the ASTC guidelines is the notion that a consultant crosses a line when he/ she becomes too directive and provide instruction regarding the content of the client's testimony. This can take the shape of suggesting answers to specific questions that are anticipated on the witness stand or urging a witness to not reveal something truthful, because it might not be beneficial to the case. Similarly, the FMHP consultant must be aware of taking too active and directive an approach in the process of "supporting" a parent through post-divorce processes.

For example, Hobbs-Minor and Sullivan (2008) accurately note the clear breach of ethics if a consultant directly assists a parent to fill out a question-naire for a custody evaluator. And, it is not unheard of for consultants to explain the MMPI-2 or the Rorschach to an anxious parent, and perhaps even preview parts of the tests, again to allay the parent's fears but which could violate the ethical rules regarding test security.

But, questions of ethics and sound professional practice arise in the grey areas. Parents often view the consultant as an authority that fills an emotional need at a time of great vulnerability. In instances where a consultant shepherds a parent-litigants through a four to six month custody evaluation, the parent is especially prone to subtle and unconscious influence. This can manifest in how parents present themselves or how they form responses during the custody evaluation. For example, take the case of an attorney and consultant working with a narcissistic parent. Many narcissistic indivi-duals are exceptionally good performers and are skilled at taking direction for impression management if doing so meets their needs and goals. However, by definition, narcissistic people also lack empathy, a quality that

Situation	Dilemma	Guidance toward solution
FMHP is hired by attorney to help "manage" an anxious parent/litigant during a CCE. The parent asks the FMHP for advice re: what to say to the evaluator that would be convincing re: her belief that she's been the victim of domestic violence.	What is needed to help the parent bind their anxiety? There may well be a pull to support the parent's perception of self as a victim that could influence the degree of "guidance" the FMHP provides. At what point would a FMHP unduly influence the CCE process?	Support can be generic without affirming whether DV has occurred; the FMHP can emphasize the limits of the information the consultant has and inability to come to a conclusion about possible DV; the consultant must be careful not to actively shape the parent's interviews with the evaluator.
FMHP is hired by attorney and signs a contract. Initial retainer is paid by the attorney, but additional checks for services start to come from the parent/litigant.	Lack of clarity as to who is the responsible party. Possible concern about attorney work product. FMHP's ability and willingness to provide honest feedback could be negatively impacted.	It's best to establish quickly that all payments should come from the attorney.
FMPH is hired to work with an anxious or reactive parent/litigant throughout a child custody evaluation or other litigation proceedings. Parent asks for specific advice and/or information about psychological tests.	How much information is useful to contain the parent's feelings and behavior (and satisfy the retaining attorney) versus how much violates test security.	Test security trumps the parent's anxiety, some of which might be expected given the circumstances. Discussing generic information about psychological tests may be acceptable; however, reviewing test items and procedures would be ethically compromising.
FMHP is hired to work confidentially with parent/litigant through CCE. Either therapy or parenting coaching is recommended by the evaluator and ordered by the court. Parent asks FMHP to be the therapist/coach.	This represents a significant shift in roles. The shift for the FMHP is from being part of the litigation team to being a service provider to the individual.	The FMHP should decline the new role. Especially if the parenting coach must now report to the court, the previously confidential work would have to be disclosed.
FMHP is asked by attorney to write a declaration on a specific topic relevant to the litigation. Then, the attorney also asks FMHP for assistance preparing cross-examination questions of witnesses.	If the FMHP agrees to help with examination preparation, there is a shift away from being a more dispassionate expert on research and literature to an advocacy role on the litigation team. This could hurt the expert's credibility as he/she would be a declared expert subject to cross examination. Confidentiality of the examination preparation is compromised.	These multiple roles are not necessarily untenable from an ethical point of view; however the consultant's credibility as a representative of the research may be questioned. The FMHP should give strong consideration to choosing one role or another.
FMHP is hired as part of the litigation team as a confidential consultant. After immersing him/herself in the case, the consultant believes that the retaining attorney's position does not support the best interests of the child.	The FMHP may be reluctant to disagree with the retaining attorney. These cases are never black and white. There may be little time for the attorney to hire another expert.	FMHP must be true to the examination of the evidence and data they review, and to the best interests of the child. It's most helpful for the FMHP to present the strengths and weaknesses of both sides of the case to the attorney, and let the attorney decide how to use the information.

FIGURE 2 Ethical dilemmas.

is central to sound, child-centered parenting. It is not hard to imagine a consultant helping such an individual present themselves more favorably than they otherwise would in the custody evaluation. There could be via seemingly benign "tips" about the parent containing behavior that might be off-putting, or a discussion of what evaluators look for on home visits or parent-child observations. A bright narcissist is often a quick study. The risk is that the parent's "improved performance" could also obscure parenting deficiencies that would be valuable for the custody evaluator to fully appreciate. Given the evaluator's task of addressing the best interest of the child, is the consultant's work ethically flawed? Have noble intentions morphed into too much advocacy? Again, these are complex issues that do not lend themselves to "bright line" interpretations.

So again, what can we "take away" that is relevant to including parents in the consulting process? The FMHP might be wise to consider the following:

- At the onset of consulting work, the FMHP should clarify with the attorney the nature and extent of anticipated contact with the parent/client. There should be an open and ongoing discussion of any possible role conflicts, especially if the consultant-parent involvement changes during the course of the attorney-consultant collaboration;
- The FMHP and attorney should clarify at the onset specifically whether the parent is expected or is likely to be a witness in a custody proceeding;
- When consultation includes direct work with a parent, the FMHP should provide informed consent to the parent, including possible limits to confidentiality. This is best done as a discussion that includes the attorney;
- If the parent will or may be a witness, the FMHP might be well advised to avoid substantive contact with the parent outside the presence of the attorney;
- If meeting with a parent prior to trial, even in the presence of the attorney, the consulting expert should uphold ethical standards including:
  - advocating that the parent/litigant tell the truth;
  - avoiding shaping or exerting undue influence on the parent's participation in a custody evaluation or legal proceedings;
  - operating within the bounds of the consultant's competence and experience;
  - reviewing the actual or potential limits on confidentiality; and
  - respecting psychological test security.

Applications in Professional Practice

What follows in Figure 2 are some examples of murkier situations the FMHP family law consultant might find him/herself in with suggestions of how to think through dilemmas these circumstances pose.

AND SO WHERE ARE WE GOING?

Working in family law and child custody can be both enormously gratifying, but equally challenging. Arguably, no other area of psychology requires the breadth and depth of skills and knowledge. At the same time, the demands are great, the stakes are very high and the venue is permeated with intense and conflicting emotions. Expanding consulting services are emanating from the increased collaborations between FMHPs and attorneys as well as the wealth of scientifically based research of the impact of divorce on children, parents, and family systems. But, concurrently, we are venturing into territory where ethical and responsible professional behavior is less well defined. This does not mean we should not be venturing, but it does mean we should be doing it thoughtfully, with open discussion of the predicaments we face, and with an eye towards constantly defining and redefining what ethical behavior is. This is what has been happening historically in the worlds of forensic psychology and trial consulting. Considerable progress has been made. The work must continue.

It would seem like a glaring omission not to re-emphasize that as FMHP working in family law, we always bear responsibility to the best interests of children. The best interests standing itself is hardly an absolute, as it involves balancing the interests of the child, the parent, and sometimes even the state as *parens patriae* (Smoron, 1998). Even the most responsible consultants, who are answerable to multiple clients and must be responsive to their own professional ethics while accommodating the rules of the legal profession, must also strive to understand the best interests of the child. It is one thing for a consultant to beg off a case where he/she has been asked to review a custody evaluation when the consultant cannot support the position of the attorney who wants to hire him/her. In a sense, that is an easy call. What is more difficult is for the FMHP consultant to not get so swept up in meeting the needs of the attorney and the parent that some understanding of what is best for children is lost in the mix. Responsible consultants owe it to all of the participants to take the time to understand this to the extent possible.

And what advice can we offer the theoretical consultant in the vignette that opened this article? While there might not be one "right way" to address the situation, there are enough warning signs to suggest that the consultant should proceed thoughtfully and with caution. He/she might be well advised to take the time needed to understand the case in the depth that it warrants, tease out the separate needs of the attorney and the parent, and delineate how the consultant can and cannot be helpful. The consultant should have the courage to ask tough questions, offer the full range of his/her thoughts and impressions, and rely on the independence and integrity of his/her professional opinions and responsibilities.

REFERENCES

Ake v. Oklahoma, 470 U.S. 68 (1985).

American Bar Association. (1983). Model rules of professional conduct. Retrieved from http://www.abanet.org/cpr/mrpc/,rpc_toc.html

American Psychological Association (APA). (1953). *Ethical standards of psychologists*. Washington, DC: Author.

American Psychological Association (APA). (1959). Ethical standards of psychologists. *American Psychologist, 14*, 279–282. doi:10.1037/h0048469

American Psychological Association (APA). (1992). Ethical standards of psychologists and code of conduct. *American Psychologist, 47*, 1597–1611. doi:10.1037/0003-066X.47.12.1597

American Psychological Association (APA). (1994). Guidelines for child custody evaluations in divorce proceedings. *American Psychologist, 47*, 1597–1611.

American Psychological Association (APA). (2002). Ethical principles of psychologists and code of conduct. *American Psychologist, 57*, 1060–1073. doi:10.1037/0003-066X.57.12.1060

Association of Family and Conciliation Courts. (2006). Model standards of practice for child custody evaluation. *Family Court Review, 45*(1), 70–91.

Beck, A., Holtzworth-Munroe, A., D'Onofrio, B., Fee, W., & Hill, F. (2009). Collaboration between judges and social science researchers in family law. *Family Court Review, 47*(3), 451–467. doi:10.1111/j.1744-1617.2009.01267.x

Beggs, G. (1995). Novel expert evidence in federal civil rights litigation. *The American University Law Review, 45*. Retrieved from http://www.wcl.american.edu/journal/lawrev/45/beggstxt.html

Brewer, N., Williams, K., & Semmler, C. (2005). Psychology and Law Research: An Overview. In N. Brewer & K. Williams (Eds.) *Psychology and law: An empirical perspective* (pp. 1–10). New York: The Guilford Press.

Briggs v. Elliott et al., 342 U.S. 350 (1952).

Brodsky, S. L. (1999). *The expert witness: More maxims and guidelines for testifying in court*. Washington, DC: American Psychological Association.

Brodsky, S. L. (2009). *Principles and practice of trial consultation*. New York: The Guilford Press.

Brown v. Board of Education of Topeka, 347 U.S. 483, 745 Ct/686, 98 L.Ed. 873 (1954).

Committee on Ethical Guidelines for Forensic Psychologists. (1991). Specialty guidelines for forensic psychologists. *Law and Human Behavior, 15*, 655–665. doi:10.1007/BF01065858

Daubert v. Merrell Dow Pharmaceuticals, Inc. (1993). 509 U.S. 579, 589.

Drogin, Eric Y. (2007). The forensic psychologist as consultant: Examples from a jurisprudent science perspective. *Journal of Psychiatry & Law, 35*(3).

Drogin, E. Y., & Barrett, C. L. (2007). Off the witness stand: The forensic psychologist as consultant. In A. M. Goldstein (Ed.) *Forensic psychology: Emerging topics and expanding roles* (pp. 465–488). Hoboken, NJ: Wiley.

Frye v. United States, Federal Reports 293 (1923), 1013–1014.

Goldstein, A. (2003). Overview of forensic psychology. In A. M. Goldstein (Ed.) *Handbook of forensic psychology* (pp. 3–20). Hoboken, NJ: Wiley.

Goldstein, A. (2007). Forensic psychology: Toward a standard of care. In A. M. Goldstein (Ed.) *Forensic psychology: Emerging topics and expanding roles* (pp. 3–41). Hoboken, NJ: Wiley.

Goodman-Delahunty, J. (1997). Forensic psychological expertise in the wake of Daubert. *Law and Human Behavior, 21*(2), 121–140. doi:10.1023/A:1024874228425

Gould, J. (1998). *Conducting scientifically crafted child custody evaluations.* Thousand Oaks, Sage Press.

Gould, J. W., Kirkpatrick, H. D., Austin, W. G., & Martindale, D. (2004). A framework and protocol for providing a forensic work product review: Application to child custody evaluations. *Journal of Child Custody: Research, Issues, and Practices, 1*(3), 37–64. doi:10.1300/J190v01n03_04

Gould, J. W., & Martindale, D. A. (2007). *The art and science of child custody evaluations.* New York: Guilford.

Greenberg, S., & Shuman, D. (2007). When worlds collide: Therapeutic and forensic roles. *Professional Psychology: Research and Practice, 38*(2), 129–132. doi:10.1037/0735-7028.38.2.129

Greenberg, S. A., & Shuman, D. W. (1997). Irreconcilable conflict between therapeutic and forensic roles. *Professional Psychology: Research and Practice, 28*, 50–57. doi:10.1037/0735-7028.28.1.50

Greenberg, S. A., Shuman, D. W., & Meyer, R. G. (2004). Unmaking forensic diagnosis. *International Journal of Law and Psychiatry, 27*, 1–15. doi:10.1016/j.ijlp.2004.01.001

Guilmette, T. J., & Hagan, L. D. (1997). Ethical considerations in forensic neuropsychological consultation. *The Clinical Neuropsychologist, 11*, 287–290. doi:10.1080/13854049708400457

Haney, C. (1982). Criminal justice and the nineteenth-century paradigm. *Law and Human Behavior, 6*, 191–235.

Heilbrun, K. (2001). *Principles of forensic mental health assessment.* New York: Kluwer Academic/Plenum Publishers.

Hickman v. Taylor, 329 U.S. 495 (1947).

Hobbs-Minor, E. (1998, Summer). Parenting plan advisor: A new role for divorce professionals. *Family Mediation News*, pp. 10–11.

Hobbs-Minor, E., & Sullivan, M. (2008). Mental health consultation in child custody cases. In L. Fieldstone & C. Coates (Eds.) *Innovations in interventions with high conflict families* (pp. 159–186). Madison: Association of Family and Conciliation Courts.

Huss, M. (2001). Psychology *and law, now and in the next century: the promise of an emerging area of psychology.* In J. Halonen & S. Davis *The many faces of psychological research in the 21st century. Society for the teaching of psychology.* Retrieved from hppt://teachpsych.org/resources/e-books/faces/index_faces.php.

In re: Cendant Corp Sec. Litig., 343 F.3d 658 (3rd Cir. 2003).

Jenkins v. United States, 307 F.2d 637 (1962).

Jones, J. L., & Mehr, S. L. (2007). Foundations and assumptions of the scientist-practitioner model. *American Behavioral Scientist, 50*(6), 766–771. doi:10.1177/0002764206296454

Kairys, D. (2008). *Philadelphia freedom: Memoir of a civil rights lawyer.* Ann Arbor: University of Michigan Press.

Kelly, R., & Ramsey, S. (2007). Assessing and communicating social science information in family and child judicial settings: Standards for judges and allied professionals. *Family and Conciliation Courts Review, 45*(1), 22–41. doi:10.1111/j.1744-1617.2007.00126.x

Kovera, M., Dickinson, J., & Cutler, B. (2003). Voir dire and jury selection. In A. M. Goldstein (Ed.) *Handbook of forensic psychology* (pp. 161–175). Hoboken, NJ: Wiley.

Levett, L., Danielsen, E., Kovera, M., & Cutler, B. (2005). The psychology of jury and juror decision making. In N. Brewer & K. Williams (Eds.) *Psychology and law: An empirical perspective* (pp. 365–406). New York: The Guilford Press.

Lewis, E. (2010). Witness preparation: What is ethical and what is not. *Litigation, 36*(2), 41–56.

Lieberman, J. D., & Sales, B. D. (2007). *Scientific jury selection.* Washington, DC: American Psychological Association. doi:10.1037/11498-000

Lipsitt, P. D. (2007). Ethics and forensic psychological practice. In A. M. Goldstein (Ed.) *Forensic psychology: Emerging topics and expanding roles* (pp. 171–189). Hoboken, NJ: Wiley.

Marston, W. (1917). Systolic blood pressure systems of deception. *Journal of Experimental Psychology, 2*(2), 117–163. doi:10.1037/h0073583

Martindale, D. A. (2006). Consultants and further role delineation. *The Matrimonial Strategist, 24,* 4, 4ff.

Münsterberg, H. (1906). *Psychology and crime.* New York: Doubleday.

Münsterberg, H. (1908). On the witness stand: Essays on psychology and crime. Retrieved March 1, 2009 from York University Web site: http://psychclassics. yorku.ca/Munster/Witness/

Münsterberg, H. (1909). *Psychotherapy.* New York: Moffat Yard. doi:10.1037/10543-000

Münsterberg, H. (1914). *Psychology and social sanity.* London: T. F. Unwin.

Nicholson, R. A., & Norwood, S. (2000). The quality of forensic psychological assessments, reports, and testimony: Acknowledging the gap between promise and practice. *Law and Human Behavior, 24*(1), 2000. doi:10.1023/A:1005422702678

Ogloff, J., & Finkelman, D. (1999). Psychology and law: An overview. In R. Roesch, S. Hart & J. Ogloff (Eds.) *Psychology and law: The state of the discipline.* New York: Kluwer Academic Press.

Perrott, D., & Wolfe, D. (2010). Out and proud; Ethical and legal considerations in retaining a trial consultant to assist with witness preparation. *The Jury Expert, January 2010;* 53–62.

Pickar, D. (2007). Countertransference bias in the child custody evaluator. *Journal of Child Custody, 4*(3/4), 45–68.

Posey, A., & Wrightsman, L. (2005). *Trial consulting.* Oxford: University Press.

RAND Institute for Criminal Justice. (2002). *Changes in the standards for admitting expert evidence.* Research brief. Retrieved from http://www.rand.org/pubs/research_briefs/RB9037/index1.html

Shuman, D. W., & Greenberg, S. A. (2003). The expert witness, the adversary system, and the voice of reason: Reconciling impartiality and advocacy. *Professional*

Psychology: Research and Practice, 34(3), 219–224. doi:10.1037/0735-7028.34.3.219

Shuman, D. W., & Sales, B. (1998). The Admissibility of expert testimony based upon clinical judgment and scientific research. *Psychology, Public Policy and the Law, 4*(4), 1226–1252. doi:10.1037/1076-8971.4.4.1226

Smoron, K. A. (1998). Conflicting roles in child custody mediation: Impartiality/ Neutrality and the best interests of the child. *Family and Conciliation Courts Review, 36*(2), 258–280. doi:10.1111/j.174-1617.1998.tb00508.x

Stahl, P. (1996). Second opinions: An ethical and professional process for reviewing child custody evaluations. *Family and Conciliation Courts Review, 34*, 386–395. doi:10.1111/j.174-1617.1996.tb00428.x

Strier, F. (1999). Whither trial consulting? Issues and projections. *Law and Human Behavior, 23*(1), 93–115. doi:10.1023/A:1022378824280

The Professional Code of the American Society of Trial Consultants (ASTC). (2008).

United States Department of Justice; Office of Information Policy. (1983). *Attorney Work-Product Protection*, FOIA Update; *IV*(3).

Weissman, H. N., & DeBow, D. M. (2003). Ethical principles and professional competencies. In A. M. Goldstein (Ed.) *Handbook of forensic psychology* (pp. 33–53). Hoboken, NJ: Wiley.

Wigmore, J. H. (1913). *Principles of judicial proof as given by logic, psychology, and general experience and illustrated in judicial trials*. Boston: Little, Brown.

Testifying Experts and Non-Testifying Trial Consultants: Appreciating the Differences

JONATHAN GOULD

Forensic Psychology Private Practice, Charlotte, North Carolina

DAVID MARTINDALE

Forensic Psychology Private Practice, St. Petersburg, Florida

TIMOTHY TIPPINS

Attorney, Albany, New York

JEFF WITTMANN

Forensic Psychology Private Practice, Albany, New York

While the roles of trial consultant and testifying expert witness share many functions, the field of forensic psychology has evolved and it appears that, among those who offer these services regularly, there is a developing consensus that keeping these roles distinct is beneficial for the forensic practitioner, for attorneys advocating for clients, for the courts, and for litigants themselves.

The forensic mental health field has evolved in complexity and breadth over the last three decades in theoretical models, empirical research, and professional practice. Within the forensic mental health field, there has been a concomitant evolution in the subspecialty of child custody assessment. The child custody professional practice literature continues to describe changes in roles and to emphasize the importance of differentiating between roles with demands that may create conflicts.

The first of the elucidated role distinctions was one between therapeutic and forensic roles. In their seminal article, Greenberg and Shuman (1997) described the irreconcilable differences between the role of the treatment provider and the role of the forensic evaluator. Weissman and DeBow (2003) have also identified several forensic mental health roles beyond that of the evaluating expert.

In this article, we limit our discussion to experts who may testify and experts employed only for trial preparation. Our decision to limit our discussion in this manner is based upon the areas of expert involvement found in Federal Rule of Civil Procedure 26. Although custody proceedings are conducted in state courts where the Federal Rules of Evidence do not apply per se, many states have modeled their evidence codes on the Federal Rules of Evidence. Common law states, such as New York, that operate in the absence of a comprehensive statutory evidence system, have generated decisional law analogs that closely parallel the Federal Rules of Evidence. Thus, the Federal Rules present a medial representation of the law of evidence even though individual states have modified them. Likewise, most states have procedural codes that parallel, though are not identical to, the Federal Rules of Civil Procedure. Obviously, with respect to both procedural and evidentiary rules, practitioners are obligated to familiarize themselves with the rules that are applicable in the jurisdictions in which they practice.

Rule 26 (b) (4) identifies the expert who may testify and the expert employed only for trial preparation. No other expert roles are described in Rule 26 and we limit our discussion to the importance of maintaining role distinctions between the expert who testifies and the expert employed to assist in trial preparation. Rather than using the terms used in the FRP 26 that refer to these roles using the word "expert," we draw a distinction between the *expert witness role,* in which it is expected at the time of being retained that the expert will be asked to present under oath a psychological opinion to the court, and a *trial consultant role,* in which it is expected at the time of being retained that the expert will not be asked to testify at trial. In this paper we present a first step in building a model for the forensic mental health professional (FMHP) engaged in consultation the purpose of which is to assist family law attorneys in preparing for trial.

Among the generally accepted *non-testifying consultant* roles are an expert hired to (1) review a work product and write direct and cross examination questions; (2) present research to the retaining attorney or litigant for educational purposes; (3) assist in identifying the psychological elements involved in the legal strategy; and (4) assist in case conceptualization, preparation, and presentation.

Several authors have written about the roles that mental health professionals may play in the legal system that are not directly related to the roles of expert witness and trial consultant as we define them in the following. We recognize that forensic mental health professionals may become involved in child custody cases as therapists for one or more children, either parent, or the family system. We acknowledge that forensic mental health professionals may consult with attorneys' clients in witness preparation, educating parents about current behavioral science literature, or other behind the scene activities that are only indirectly related to the task of trial preparation. Greenberg and her colleagues have written about the need to differentiate between a treating expert and a forensic expert (Greenberg & Gould, 2001; Greenberg, Gould, Gould-Saltman, & Stahl, 2004; Greenberg, Martindale, Gould, & Gould-Saltman, 2004; Greenberg, Gould, Gould-Saltman, & Stahl, 2003; Greenberg, Gould, Schnider, Gould-Saltman, & Martindale, 2003). "The essential characteristic of the treating psychologist's role, as distinguished from the child custody evaluator, is that the goal is intervention. The purpose of a child custody evaluator is to gather information to answer specific questions about the family's functioning (e.g., parenting competencies or the child's safety with either parent)" (p. 473). Other authors have written about mental health consultation to attorneys that includes, but is not limited to, educating attorneys about current literature, and advising parents about application of behavioral science research regarding child development to their particular case (Ackerman & Kane, 2004; Gould, 2006).

Among the generally accepted *testifying expert witness roles* that are accepted in courts today are (1) court appointed, neutral evaluator; (2) case-blind didactic expert, who only provides information about research without having reviewed any case related documents; (3) testifying, evaluating expert hired by one side to conduct an evaluation; and (4) work product reviewer, hired by one side, who, after having completed a review, testifies to his/her assessment of the work reviewed.

NOT ALL HIRED GUNS SHOOT STRAIT

Let us not ignore the 800-pound gorilla in the room. Experts who have been retained by one side are often disparagingly referred to as "hired guns." However, FMHPs who are retained by one side in a custody dispute are not necessarily snake oil salesmen who eagerly sell their souls for a buck. Many of us who are retained by one side in a legal dispute practice in a manner consistent with ethical codes of conduct and professional practice guidelines for forensic psychologists. There is an important distinction between principled FHMPs retained by one side in a legal dispute and unprincipled FMHPs. Unprincipled FMH experts will testify to any opinion that someone pays them to testify to, will cite research that they know to be flawed, and will be unconcerned that they are misleading judges. Providing biased, advocacy based testimony is a violation of the oath to "tell the whole truth and nothing but the truth." We do not take an oath to tell only the part of the truth that fits the story to be told by one side in the litigation. Expert witnesses swear to tell the whole truth.

Principled FMH experts are knowledgeable and familiar with applicable research; able to discern the difference between sound methodology and flawed methodology; able to interpret test data without computer-generated interpretive reports; and, have formulated opinions on various issues based upon their studies. Inevitably, there will be times when an opinion held by the FMHP is precisely the opinion that a particular attorney wants a judge to hear. When the principled expert is paid to come to court and explain that opinion to the judge, the expert is being paid for time expended and nothing more. The principled retained expert takes seriously the most basic obligation of an expert witness: the obligation to assist the court.

Some colleagues are critical of the distinction we draw between testifying expert and trial consultant. They seem to reject the notion that a testifying expert who reviews a work product is unable to maintain the cognitive and emotional distance needed to minimize alignment with the legal position of the attorney who has retained them. They also have called into question our belief that judges will view our work as less biased when testifying experts minimize contact with the retaining attorney prior to formulating their opinions about the work products being reviewed.

Ramsey and Kelly (2009) draw a distinction between a non-party advocacy brief and a state of the scientific knowledge brief. "Non-party advocacy briefs typically argue for the ethical, political, or policy interests of the filing organization or individual. Briefs such as these are generally expected to take an advocacy position, and it is acceptable for them to emphasize information that supports their viewpoint and to deemphasize information that does not" (p. 83). State of the scientific knowledge briefs purport to present "an objective summary of social science research that is relevant to the legal issues the court is considering" (p. 83). Input provided by experts retained to conduct work product reviews should be similar to the input contained in state of the science knowledge amicus briefs. Reviewers' comments should be fair, even handed, objective, and reflect an objective appraisal of the methods and procedures used in the assessment, an objective appraisal of the comprehensiveness of literature reviewed in the body of the report, and a fair-minded analysis of the relationship between the data and the opinions generated by those data. We do not believe that the role of the reviewer is to advocate for a particular legal position as is reflected in the description of a non-party advocacy brief.

Some colleagues who reviewed our drafts of this article believed our position to be naïve. Their arguments were that (a) attorneys do not retain testimonial experts without first having determined that the testimony to be offered will support the attorneys' legal position and (b) retained experts face considerable financial and personal pressure to please those who have retained. Addressing the first concern, it is irrefutable that competent attorneys will only retain as expert witnesses those experts whose positions are likely to support the attorneys' legal positions. That does not mean that the experts who sign on have tailored their findings and opinions to meet the needs of the retaining attorneys. In the model endorsed by us, FMHPs utilize two separate and distinctly different contracts. The first contract sets forth the terms under which a work product review will be conducted. At the conclusion of their work product reviews, FMHPs employing this model orally communicate their findings and opinions to the attorneys who have retained them. When those findings and opinions are not what the retaining attorneys had hoped to hear, the attorneys and experts usually part company and the involvement of the experts is, more often than not, undisclosed. When the findings and opinions orally imparted by the experts to the attorneys are viewed by the attorneys as supportive of their legal positions, the FMHPs employing this model then offer either to provide litigation support services *or* to offer testimony.

We are not naïve concerning the potentially pernicious effect of retention bias: the desire to please those from whom remuneration flows. It is our view, however, that the negative impact of retention bias on the delivery of helpful expert testimony by retained FMHPs is overestimated. Dr. Flexible, a FMHP who expresses opinion A when retained by Attorney A and expresses opposing opinion B when retained by Attorney B is likely to be identified as a FMHP whose objective is to please those who are paying the bill rather than to assist the trier of fact.

Peer Review as Exemplar

As indicated previously, in the model endorsed by us, both testimonial services and litigation support services begin with an oral, rather than written, presentation to the attorney of the findings and opinions of the FMHP. If reviewers are subsequently identified as testimonial experts, findings and opinions that have been memorialized in writing are likely to be subject to disclosure during the course of the pre-trial discovery process. Initial findings and opinions may undergo significant changes as reviewers gather and review information that was unavailable at the time of the initial review. As reviewers obtain raw data and contemporaneously-taken notes (likely not to have been available at the time of the initial review), their views of the evaluative methodology, the data analyses, and the nexus between data gathered and opinions expressed may undergo modification. Though MHPs tend to view favorably the ability of colleagues to modify preliminary opinions when exposed to new information, modified opinions are viewed as pre-holiday gifts to cross-examining attorneys.

Reviewing FMHPs should not presume that they have sufficient knowledge of the rules of discovery to make decisions that are likely to have implications for the discovery process. It is preferable that the written contractual agreement under the terms of which a work product review is conducted should be separate from any subsequent contractual agreement either for testimonial services or for litigation support services.

It is only after having received oral input from retained reviewers that attorneys can make informed decisions concerning whether or not further services are desired and, if so, whether those services should be testimonial or consultative. If the post-review service to be rendered by a FMHP will involve formal communication with the court, either by means of a written report or by means of oral testimony, the FMHP should limit his/her statements to those that conform to the admonitions that appear in Standards 2.04 and 9.01 (a) of the Psychologists' Ethics Code, in Model Standard 12.3 of the AFCC's Model Standards for Child Custody Evaluation, and in Guideline VI. H. of the Specialty Guidelines for Forensic Psychologists.

Work Product Commentary and Second Opinions

The field of forensic psychology has changed considerably over the past two decades. For example, in 1996, Stahl, in an article addressing work product reviews, made reference to "a second opinion, either with a new evaluation, or with a review of the original evaluation in order to show the judge that the recommendations in the original evaluation should not be followed" (Stahl, 1996). Information gathered by FMHPs retained by one side in an adversarial proceeding is, by its very nature, insufficient and skewed. For this reason, it cannot be viewed as information sufficient to form the basis for opinions relating to the issues in dispute. Reviewers offering testimony should limit their opinions to matters concerning the manner in which the reviewed evaluation was performed.

We have written elsewhere that the use of the term "second opinion" is incorrect as it is used in this context. A second opinion is a second evaluation that generates sufficient data upon which to offer a reliable second opinion. A review examines the methodology of an evaluation (Gould, Kirkpatrick, Austin, & Martindale, 2004). It is not a new evaluation.

Even the most diligent and skilled reviewer cannot gather information that is quantitatively and qualitatively sufficient to form the basis for opinions concerning the issues in dispute. FMHPs who perform work product reviews and who, subsequently, testify or file reports for courts concerning their reviews should limit the opinions expressed to matters relating to the work that has been reviewed (or to opinions about broad psychological principles or hypothetical questions) and should exercise care not to opine on the issues of (a) the psychological functioning of the litigants or their children, or of (b) custodial placement and access for the family in question.

An exception may be made when an admissible hypothetical question is posed to an expert witness. When this is done, included in the formulation of the question are all of the pertinent facts in evidence that would be reasonably needed in order for the expert to formulate an opinion that can be expressed with a reasonable degree of professional certainty. There is a critical difference between a response offered to a hypothetical question (even though it is clear to all that the question pertains to an issue in dispute or party to the litigation) and specific opinions offered about named individuals who have not been evaluated. The difference is that if the hypothetical question, as framed by the questioner, is felt by opposing counsel to assume facts not in evidence; to misrepresent facts in evidence; or, to omit facts that, if included, might reasonably be expected to alter the opinion offered by the testifying witness, opposing counsel can object to the hypothetical as framed.

Testimony by reviewing experts is most effective when experts are perceived by the court to have a genuine interest in educating judges concerning good methodology, flawed methodology, and the ways in which methodological errors can lead evaluators to make misguided recommendations. If experts who are endeavoring to educate judges regarding methodological flaws in evaluations are asked on cross-examination whether they have met with or discussed the case with any of the interested parties, the usefulness of the experts' testimony is dependent upon their responses. Just as evaluators must employ sound methodology or face the consequences of not having done so when they encounter a skilled cross-examining attorney, so too must reviewers employ sound methodology or face well-deserved jabs at their credibility during cross-examination. Experts who have had contact with litigants, family members, or allies are likely to be perceived as less objective, as less devoted to sound methodology, and, therefore, as less credible.

It is not possible to meet with individuals without forming impressions of them and such impressions may impair reviewers' objectivity as they endeavor to focus on methodology. We recognize that threats to reviewer objectivity cannot be completely avoided. Objectivity is not a dichotomous variable. Objectivity is a mental state to be sought, even as we recognize that absolute objectivity is unattainable. For example, even when serving as a peer reviewer, it is more and more common for FMHP's to be presented with family videos taken by litigants. Reviewers examining evaluators' files will find themselves forming impressions of the litigants as they inspect these videos. We conceptualize this as one of the unavoidable threats to objectivity. Our awareness of this threat to objectivity does not alter our perspective on the importance of guarding against those threats to objectivity that *are* avoidable.

Awards for Professional Courtesy

When the awards for professional courtesy are being handed out, reviewers will not be among the recipients. In discussing work product review procedures, Stahl (1996) stated that the reviewer should "talk with the evaluator . . ." in order to be able to demonstrate that the reviewer has "considered the evaluator's position through the evaluator's eyes before reaching a different conclusion (p. 389)." We offer a different perspective: After having completed a work product review, before offering the first critical comment about the evaluator's work, walk a mile in his shoes. This ensures that if the evaluator is angered by your critical comments, you are a mile away and you have his shoes.

Another change that has taken place in the field over the past 20 years is seen in Stahl-2010's disagreement with Stahl-1996. In 1996, Stahl emphasized that "the review must adequately blend a process of listening to the evaluator and understanding the evaluator's process and conclusions while providing an educational and didactic component that teaches the evaluator what the reviewer believes was missing in the original evaluation (p. 393)." We are in disagreement with Stahl's original position, as is Stahl, himself (personal communication, October 5, 2010. Quoted with permission. Original e-mail on file). It is our position, and now Stahl's himself, that reviewers should not communicate with those whose work they are reviewing. The authority to decide whether or not reviewers should communicate with those whose work is under review rests with the retaining attorney and not with the reviewer. Only rarely would a retaining attorney wish that such communication to take place.

There are two additional reasons why reviewers should not communicate with those whose work is under review. If the retained reviewer is a trial consultant, her role is to assist the attorney in preparing for trial. The non-testimonial consultant is working as an extension of the attorney and, therefore, any communication between the retained consultant and the court appointed evaluator may be viewed as an ex parte communication. The retained consultant's responsibility is to share all information and opinions with the attorney. Any conversations between the retained consultant and the court appointed evaluator would be viewed as the court appointed evaluator providing information directly to one side in the case. The retained consultant has no obligation to share with opposing counsel any information obtained in conversations with the court appointed evaluator, possibly compromising the balance of fairness in the adjudicative process.

Second, discussions between reviewers and evaluators bring to the review process information that is not part of the record and, for that reason, leads to problems that cannot be ignored. Explanations offered orally by evaluators to reviewers concerning the bases for the evaluators' expressed opinions are explanations that should appear in their reports and, subsequently, in their testimony. Decisions concerning the adequacy of such explanations must be made by the parties during pre-trial settlement endeavors and by the court if the case proceeds to trial. An explanation offered orally to a reviewer is not a suitable substitute for an explanation incorporated into an evaluator's written discussion of the bases for opinions expressed and is certainly no substitute for a rationale offered under oath.

The Case for Role Differentiation

The case law foundation for the difference between a testifying expert and a non-testifying consultant was addressed in *Ake v. Oklahoma* [470 U.S. 68

(1985)]. In *Ake*, the U.S. Supreme Court noted the need for a litigant to have access to a non-testimonial consultant whose tasks might include assisting in the preparation of trial related materials such as direct and cross examination questions.

The *Ake* decision helped elucidate the role of the FMHP as trial consultant. In this role, the FMHP provides assistance to a legal team in developing its theory of the case; identifying deficiencies in the testimony of expert witnesses who weaken the team's case, including inadequacies in their professional backgrounds, investigative methods and procedures; exploring the manner in which research has been utilized and described; and, commenting on the degree to which the opinions offered in written and/or oral testimony are supported by the data generated in the evaluation.

A testifying expert's role is to inform the court. *The Specialty Guidelines for Forensic Psychologists* (Committee on Ethical Guidelines for Forensic Psychologists, 1991) admonish testifying psychologists to advocate for the data and not to advocate for a litigation position. A non-testimonial consultant may, through his or her crafting of direct or cross examination questions, assist an attorney, whose ethical responsibility is to "zealously advocate" for the litigant's legal position, thereby assisting in the advocacy for a specific litigation position.

It is our position that participating in the role of a testimonial expert witness and simultaneously functioning as a behind the scenes trial consultant to a legal team represents a dual role. One cannot advocate for the data if at the same time one is being asked to advocate for a legal position. Heilbrun, testifying as the State's expert in *Jan C. Grossman v. State Board of Psychology* [No. 3023 C. D. (2001)], has questioned the ethical propriety of such dual roles.

The FMHPs who testify are obligated to assist the trier of fact. When testifying FMHPs, who have presented themselves as educators to the court, are observed by the judge to be actively providing litigation support, it is likely that the judge will conclude that the earlier testimony was not as neutral and free of bias as it may have appeared.

Despite our advanced training in forensic mental health services, being human renders us susceptible to the same forces of coercion, bias, and affiliation as are individuals with less training or different professional backgrounds. Participation on a team that is advocating for a position is far more likely than not to affect how FMHPs attend to data (particularly when some data are not congruent with other data) interpret data, decide what weight to assign to different data, and integrate different sets of data with one another. When the goal of the legal team is to prevail at trial (as is always the case), active involvement by a FMHP in the competitive effort dramatically decreases the probability that the FMHP will be able to function as a dispassionate educator to the court.

Our recommendation that FMHPs function either as providers of litigation support services or as testifying experts, but not as both in the same case, is supported by research on the social and cognitive factors that influence decision making (Arkes, 1981, 1991; Borum, Otto, & Golding, 1993; Brehm & Cohen,1962; Dailey, 1952; Klayman & Ha, 1987; Koriat, Lichtenstein, & Fischhoff, 1980; Sandifer, Hordern, & Green, 1970; Sanfey, 2007; Tversky & Kahneman, 1974).

The Temptation to Combine Roles

While trial consultants have been used to assist legal teams for many decades in criminal and other areas of civil litigation, the use of trial consultants is a recent addition to the armamentarium of family law practitioners. Because of the newness of the role of trial consultant in the family law field, there has been a tendency for family law attorneys to invite testimonial experts to become involved in litigation support and to offer testimony. With no litera-ture to guide them, forensic mental health practitioners have often accepted the invitation to participate in both roles simultaneously.

The argument that, where financial constraints make it unfeasible for attorneys to retain more than one FMHP, the FMHP who is retained may function both (a) as a provider of litigation support services and (b) as a tes-timonial expert represents compromising important ethical principles in the service of a litigant's budgetary concerns. Allowing these two distinct roles to merge in attempts to be responsive to financial constraints is unwise. Func-tioning as a provider of litigation support services requires that the FMHP adopt an adversarial mind-set. Even when a FMHP has been retained by one side, when offering testimony, the obligation of the FMHP is to assist the trier of fact. The ability of a testimonial expert to assist the court is signi-ficantly compromised when the FMHP is also offering litigation support services to the retaining attorney.

Many attorneys view the distinction between a testimonial expert and a trial consultant as nonsense. An understandable retort from an attorney to a forensic expert's objection to engaging in both roles would be the following: "I expect you to be objective in either role, so what's the issue?" However, we have often found that if the two roles are clearly explained to the attorney and if the potential concerns about the impact on witness credibility and opening the door on protected communications between the legal team and the testifying expert are properly revealed, most attorneys recognize the utility of keeping these two roles separate.

When FMHPs who have been functioning as trial consultants subse-quently become testifying expert witnesses, the FMHPs, whose work as con-sultants had been protected from disclosure by work product privilege, are now likely to be discoverable by virtue of the FMHPs' designation as wit-nesses. Notes taken by these consulting FMHPs turned witnesses are likely to include ideas about trial strategy and opinions concerning soft spots in the cases of those who have retained them. The disclosure of the files of these FMHPs is likely to derail the trial strategies of those who have retained them.

It should come as no surprise that actions taken by FMHPs that have negative consequences for litigants, can, subsequently, have negative consequences for the FMHPs. A litigant whose case has been eviscerated by a FMHP's role change is likely to complain to a licensing board. In such a complaint, it would be asserted that "[w]hen assuming forensic roles, psychologists are or become reasonably familiar with the judicial or administrative rules governing their roles" [from Standard 2.01 (f)]; that, by logical extension, MHPs offering forensic services are obligated to be cognizant of "the foreseeable uses of the information gathered through their psychological activities" [from Standard 4.02 (a) (2)]; that the FMHP should have foreseen that records created while the FMHP was functioning as a consultant would become discoverable when the FMHP became an identified witness; and, that the damage done to the litigant's legal strategy should also have been foreseen.

The Benefits of Role Distinction

Though separating testimonial and consultancy roles may create greater financial burden for litigants (since they may need to pay two experts), doing so provides substantial benefits. A non-testifying trial consultant's records are ordinarily protected from disclosure by attorney work product privilege, especially if the consultant is wise enough to insist that the attorney, not the litigant, be identified as the consultant's client. Within the context of an attorney-consultant relationship (the records of which are not subject to discovery demands) an open, candid, and unfiltered exchange of opinions can take place. In this context, the FMHP trial consultant and the legal team can discuss the strengths and weaknesses of the team's legal position and can explore ways in which published research in the mental health fields might enable the team to construct a stronger legal argument.

When testifying FMHPs offer litigation support services tactical problems are created. Discussions between the testifying FMHPs and the attorneys who have retained them are more likely than not to be subject to discovery demands. Exchanges of information and perspectives that have taken place in written form may have to be disclosed and the disclosure may be disadvantageous. Even if such exchanges have been oral, FMHPs who have been identified as testimonial experts are likely to be deposed and, in the course of these depositions, are likely to be required to provide their recollections of these exchanges of information and perspectives.

The expert witness role is generally well understood and well defined both in law and in psychology. In custody and access matters it includes such functions as neutral evaluations of families or individuals, with opinions subsequently communicated in testimony; peer reviews of the professional work products of other clinicians, opinions subsequently offered in court; and, summaries for the court of academic literature on particular topics (i.e., case-blind didactic testimony).

The trial consultant role can involve, but is not limited to the following: (1) record review with forensic opinion; (2) assistance with case conceptualization; (3) crafting of direct and cross examination questions; (4) identification of appropriate expert witnesses; (5) expert witness preparation; (6) behind the scenes feedback to attorneys about client liabilities and strengths; (7) behind the scenes feedback regarding case weaknesses and strengths; (8) searches of the professional literature and provision of summaries on specific topics; (9) development of responses to foreseeable strategies of opposing counsel; (10) review forensic work products for trial preparation; and, (11) in court monitoring of testimony for the purpose of assisting in the development of direct and cross approaches.

Both the testifying expert and the consulting expert may prepare material pertaining to (1) procedural safeguards; (2) interview techniques with the parents; (3) interview techniques with the children; (4) the evaluator's observation of interpersonal interactions between parents; (5) the evaluator's observation of interpersonal interactions between children and parents; (6) the evaluator's use of pertinent documents; (7) the evaluator's use of collateral source information; (8) the evaluator's assessment of the reliability of collateral source information relied upon; (9) steps taken to corroborate information relied upon; (10) the manner in which assessment instruments were selected; (11) the manner in which assessment instruments were administered and, in particular, adherence (or lack thereof) to manual instructions; (12) the manner in which assessment data have been interpreted and whether there are indications of reliance upon computer-generated interpretive reports; (13) respect for role boundaries; and (14) the creation, maintenance, and production of appropriate records. The testifying expert may also (15) identify areas of investigative interest that were not pursued and the potential relevance of obtaining information from those unexamined areas. Both the testifying expert and the consulting expert can opine on (16) whether non-supporting data appear to have been considered by the evaluator; (17) whether rival hypotheses appear to have been considered; (18) whether consideration was given to pertinent statutes and case law; and (19) whether there exist indicators of examiner bias. Indicators of evaluator bias include (1) the application of a double standard; (2) the use of insulting or demeaning terminology in describing the non-favored parent; (3) the use of idealizing terminology in describing the favored parent; (4) the assignment of minimal importance to possible parenting deficiencies in the favored parent; (5) the assignment of special importance to reported flaws in the non-favored parent; (6) the seemingly wholesale acceptance of the favored parent's perspective; and (7) the seemingly wholesale rejection of the non-favored parent's perspective.

Both types of forensic consultants can offer commentary on the manner in which evaluators have communicated their findings and opinions. Specifically, consultants can opine on (1) whether information reasonably needed by the court has been included; (2) whether personal perspectives have been shared with the court in the guise of professional opinions; (3) whether known limitations in methods or data have been acknowledged; (4) whether non-supporting data have been included; (5) whether assessment data have been presented in a manner that is balanced and understandable to non-psychologists; and (6) whether the criteria employed in examining the "best interests" standard have been articulated. Articulation of such criteria is of particular importance in jurisdictions in which these are neither statutorily defined nor alluded to in case law.

Although both forensic consultants may review a work product in similar ways, the testifying expert prepares for trial by studying the materials provided by the evaluator and his or her own critique of that evaluation. The testifying expert's primary concern is communicating to the court information and opinions about the methodological integrity of the evaluation. The consulting expert prepares for trial by becoming an integral part of the legal team, developing legal strategy and helping the legal team in *its* efforts to win.

When the recipient of one's observations and opinions is a retaining attorney, it is legitimate, in the role of the consultant, to share any notions that might be helpful to that attorney—including clinical insights, hunches, theories, and premonitory visions. By contrast, when the recipient of one's statements is the court, there exists an obligation, in the role of the expert witness, to limit opinions to those that can be expressed with a reasonable degree of professional certainty. No reviewer, however astute, can opine appropriately on the issues before the court, and it is irresponsible to suggest otherwise.

Sound methodology increases the probability of formulating a supportable opinion, whereas deficient methodology increases the probability of formulating a flawed opinion. This is true whether one is an evaluator or a reviewer. It is the focus that is different. The evaluator is the only mental health professional who has conducted a comprehensive assessment and, therefore, has sufficient basis to opine on the issues before the court. The reviewer can only opine on the methodological sufficiency of the report; not opine on the issues before the court about the specific children, parents, and family seeking the court's assistance.

SUGGESTIONS FOR PRACTICE

We offer several suggestions for practice.

1. Attorneys should avoid asking forensic experts to take on the dual role of consultant to the legal team and testifying expert witness and FMHPs should resist engaging in such dual roles.

2. Attorneys should have an explicit, written contract with the forensic expert regarding which role s/he will be assuming with the legal team.
3. To ensure confidentiality of the expert's work, the designated "client" engaging the FMHP should be the legal team and not the litigant.

FINAL THOUGHTS

While the roles of trial consultant and testifying expert witness share many functions, the field of forensic psychology has evolved to a point where there is an emerging consensus that keeping these roles distinct is beneficial for the forensic practitioner, for attorneys advocating for clients, for the courts, and for litigants themselves.

REFERENCES

Ackerman, M. J., & Kane, A. W. (2004). *Psychological experts in divorce actions* (4th ed.). New York: Wiley.

Ake v. Oklahoma 470 U.S. 68 (1985).

Arkes, H. R. (1981). Impediments to accurate clinical judgment and possible ways to minimize their impact. *Journal of Consulting and Clinical Psychology, 49,* 323–330.

Arkes, H. R. (1991). Costs and benefits of judgment errors: Implications for debiasing. *Psychological Bulletin, 110,* 486–498.

Borum, R., Otto, R. K., & Golding, S. (1993). Improving clinical judgment and decision making in forensic evaluation. *Journal of Psychiatry and Law, 21,* 35–76.

Brehm, J. W., & Cohen, A. R. (1962). *Explorations in cognitive dissonance.* New York: Wiley.

Committee on Ethical Guidelines for Forensic Psychologists. (1991). Specialty guidelines for forensic psychologists. *Law and Human Behavior, 15*(6), 655–665.

Dailey, C. A. (1952). The effects of premature conclusions upon the acquisition of understanding of a person. *Journal of Psychology, 33,* 133–152.

Gould, J. W. (2006). *Conducting scientifically crafted child custody evaluations* (2nd ed.). Sarasota: Professional Research Press.

Gould, J. W., Kirkpatrick, H. D., Austin, W., & Martindale, D. A. (2004). Critiquing a colleague's forensic work product: A suggested protocol for application to child custody evaluations. *Journal of Child Custody, 1*(3), 37–64.

Greenberg, L. R., & Gould, J. W. (2001). The treating expert: A hybrid role with firm boundaries. *Professional Psychology: Research and Practice, 32*(5), 469–478.

Greenberg, L. R., Gould, J. W., Gould-Saltman, D. J., & Stahl, P. M. (2004). Is the child's therapist part of the problem? GPSolo. American Bar Association. Retrieved from www.abanet.org/genpractice/magazine/Sept2004/domestic.html

Greenberg, L. R., Gould, J. W., Gould-Saltman, D. J., & Stahl, P. M. (2003). Is the child's therapist part of the problem? What judges, attorneys, and mental health professionals need to know about Court-related treatment for children. *Family Law Quarterly, 3*, 241–271.

Greenberg, L. R., Gould, J. W., Schnider, R., Gould-Saltman, D. J., & Martindale, D. A. (2003, December). Effective intervention with high conflict families: How judges can recognize and promote competent treatment in family court. *Journal of the Center for Families, Children, and the Courts*, 1–18.

Greenberg, L. R., Martindale, D. A., Gould, J. W., & Gould-Saltman, D. J. (2004). Ethical issues in child custody and dependency cases: Enduring principles and emerging challenges. *Journal of Child Custody, 1*(1), 9–32.

Greenberg, S. A., & Shuman, D. W. (1997). Irreconcilable conflict between therapeutic and forensic roles. *Professional Psychology: Research & Practice, 28*, 50–57.

Jan, C. Grossman, v. State Board of Psychology. No. 3023 C. D. (2001).

Kelly, R. F., & Ramsey, S. H. (2009). Standards for social science amicus briefs in family and child law cases. *The Journal of Gender, Race, & Justice, 13*(1), 81–103.

Klayman, J., & Ha, Y.-W. (1987). Confirmation, disconfirmation, and information in hypothesis testing. *Psychological Review, 94*, 211–228.

Koriat, A., Lichtenstein, S., & Fischhoff, B. (1980). Reasons for confidence. *Journal of Experimental Psychology: Human Learning and Memory, 6*, 107–118.

Sandifer, M., Hordern, A., & Green, L. (1970). The psychiatric interview: The impact of the first three minutes. *American Journal of Psychiatry, 126*, 968–973.

Sanfey, A. G. (2007). Social decision-making: insights from game theory and neuroscience. *Science, 318*(5850), 598–602.

Stahl, P. (1996). Second opinions: An ethical and professional process for reviewing child custody evaluations. *Family and Conciliation Court Review, 34*(3), 386–395.

Tversky, A., & Kahneman, D. (1974). Judgment under uncertainty: Heuristics and biases. *Science, 185*, 1124–1131.

Weissman, H. N., & DeBow, D. M. (2003). Ethical principles and professional competencies. In A. M. Goldstein (Ed.), *Handbook of psychology, Volume 11: forensic psychology* (pp. 33–54). New York: Wiley.

Forensic Expert Roles and Services in Child Custody Litigation: Work Product Review and Case Consultation

WILLIAM G. AUSTIN

Independent Practice, Lakewood, Colorado

MILFRED D. DALE

Attorney at Law and Psychologist, Independent Practice, Topeka, Kansas

H. D. KIRKPATRICK

Independent Practice, Charlotte, North Carolina

JAMES R. FLENS

Independent Practice, Brandon, Florida

Courts determining the best interests of children in custody disputes frequently request help from mental health experts. This article addresses the three expert services typically provided to the court (evaluator, reviewer, and instructor) as well as the trial consultation services offered to attorneys for the parties. After noting recent developments in scientific methodology and processes that evaluators use to inform and instruct the court, we examine the work product review and consultation services that have emerged to help the court understand the scientific relevance and reliability of the evaluator's work product. But reviewers, instructional experts, and consultants are retained by attorneys, not the court. Ethical reviewers and consultants remain objective and loyal to the data and facts of the case. While others have suggested ethical and professional standards based upon "role" designations, we advocate for recognizing the overlapping nature of these four services and argue that reducing these services to their "role" obfuscates the complexity and multiple facets within each service. Establishing best practices and minimum standards should revolve around the expert's loyalty to the data, the ability to develop

opinions based upon this factual basis, and the ability to resist
pressures that bias or distort this process.

BEST INTERESTS OF THE CHILD AND EXPERT ROLES

The use of mental health experts and the role of science in child custody disputes face new and evolving challenges. When a child custody dispute cannot be settled informally or through mediation, and the parties have sufficient financial means, it is not uncommon for mental health experts to be involved. If a case needs to be litigated the court may appoint a custody evaluator. The evaluator will be in the role of the court's neutral expert to conduct an objective evaluation and address the issues in the case for the court. With increasing frequency attorneys are utilizing, or retaining, experts to provide trial consultation and/or to review the work product of the custody evaluator (i.e., custody report and file), and to offer testimony. Evaluators, therefore, should approach their task with in anticipation that their work product and opinions will be reviewed by a forensic expert (Austin, Kirkpatrick, & Flens, in press). A review occurs usually after a discerning attorney perceives there are potential problems with the evaluator's methodology, bias, or that the opinions do not seem to correspond with the facts and circumstances of the case.

This article addresses the consultation and work product review services that forensic mental health experts provide in custody cases. We examine the ethical issues associated with the role of a forensic consultant-reviewer in custody cases. We emphasize that reviewers have an ethical duty to be objective, balanced, and accurate in their analysis and in the formulation and communication of expert opinions, even though they are hired or retained by an attorney. A standard of practice for consultant-reviewers has not yet been developed with only a few professional publications on the review role and service (Gould, Kirkpatrick, Austin, & Martindale, 2004; Stahl, 1996; Martindale & Gould, 2008). This issue of the journal is a step toward establishing practice parameters for this emerging forensic role.

Regardless of the particular role assigned, all forensic mental health experts operate under and must be attuned to the best interests of the child legal standard (BICS). This standard is an attractive ideal requiring consideration of each individual child's developmental and psychological needs rather than presumptively accepting parental demands, societal stereotypes, and cultural traditions (Kelly, 1997). The BICS can also be framed as or transformed into a general variable or concept (Hage, 1972), and this is a necessary operation for custody evaluators who must define, measure, and demonstrate that the parenting plan recommended by the expert is likely to be either beneficial or least detrimental to the child. Prominent scholars in the fields of psychology and law have criticized the use of BICS as too vague, value-laden, and without a sufficient scientific research basis (Melton, Petrila, Poythress, & Slobogin, 2007; Emery, Otto, & O'Donahue, 2005). Nonetheless, courts with great regularity look to mental health experts and custody evaluators to provide guidance for decisions in these difficult cases. Mnookin (1975) long ago astutely observed that while the legal standard of BICS was not without its problems, it was the best alternative to guide decision makers. Kelly and Ramsey (2009) point out any general concept, such as BICS, can be theoretically defined and measured. Custody evaluators measure factors relevant to the children's adjustment and make best interest predictions in virtually every case. Austin (2009) asserts custody evaluations are an "easy target" for critics because of the complexity of the forensic task, but there is a vast research literature relevant to the issues commonly faced by custody evaluators, as well as numerous literature reviews for them to draw from (see Kelly & Emery, 2003).

All forensic experts in some way must address questions that are before the court in terms of what parenting plan will be in the child's best interests, meaning what parenting arrangements will facilitate a healthy behavioral-emotional adjustment and long-term development. A child's best interests can be thought of as reflecting or referring to the child's predicted adjustment and level of development, or the outcomes that are associated with his or her living environment, which in turn is partly determined by the parenting arrangement. When there is a child custody evaluation, the evaluator's task is to make predictions about the child's long-term outcomes on the basis of many factors that are considered. When the evaluator has to explain or defend his or her expert opinions, it is done so by identifying these important factors, or independent variables, and the supporting data on those factors. When the judge writes an opinion in the case it too must take the form of identifying the important factors and supporting evidence that will explain or justify the court-ordered parenting plan. When the reviewer enters a case he or she is advising the retaining attorney on the quality and accuracy of the evaluator's work in making a best interest analysis.

Changes in the last fifty years of child custody law and the proliferation of social science research reflect paradigm shifts and pendulum swings in the prevailing scientific and societal views of what is in the "best interests of the child (Elrod & Dale, 2008). Developments within the child custody evaluation professional community have worked to keep pace. This professional community is now working with a second generation of standards for evaluation methodology and communication (Association of Family and Conciliation Courts, 2006/2007; American Psychological Association, 1994;

2009) and is informed by second and third editions of authoritative texts (Ackerman, 2001; Gould, 2006; Gould & Martindale, 2007; Rohrbaugh, 2008; Galatzer-Levy, Kraus, & Galatzer-Levy, 2009). The result has been increasingly sophisticated approaches by custody evaluators to the best interests of the child task. The guidelines and literature help define a best practices framework for assessing the quality of a custody evaluation. It is also possible for a reviewer to use the perspective of a minimal standard of practice as well (Kirkpatrick, 2004).

Mental health professionals may now help the court by functioning as (1) an expert child custody evaluator; (2) an instructional expert witness; (3) an expert reviewer of the evaluator (i.e., reviewer); or (4) a trial consultant. This article reflects a step towards defining best practices and minimum standards for these four expert services within the context of child custody litigation. We discuss general issues involved in doing review work such as the ethics of combining case consultation with the retaining attorney and testifying as a reviewer expert. We discuss the ethical considerations involved in determining what opinions an expert can express in custody cases when he or she has not been an evaluator for the court.

We will discuss how authorities have viewed *expert roles* and take the position that it is more helpful and more consistent with the realities of forensic practice in child custody to describe and delineate the forensic *services* being provided by an expert rather than view the process of forensic mental health work in terms of discrete roles and functions. These roles and functions need to be identified, but they overlap in most cases where forensic experts are utilized (Mnookin & Gross, 2003).

EXPERT ROLES AND FORENSIC SERVICES IN CHILD CUSTODY

This is an article about the services forensic experts provide to the court and attorneys and the challenges confronted by experts who venture into the forensic arena. We are concerned only with custody cases that reach the litigation phase and involve a child custody evaluation. This is a very small percentage of divorces. The vast majority of divorcing parents informally settle their parenting issues. We will not discuss the specifics on how mental health professionals should properly conduct comprehensive child custody evaluations. The reference for best standard of practice is well defined by professional guidelines (AFCC, 2006/2007; APA, 2009) and authoritative texts (Gould, 2006; Martindale & Gould, 2007). We focus on the role of mental health experts who offer consultation to attorneys in child custody cases and the services provided by experts who are hired, or "retained," by attorneys to provide consultation on the mental health issues in the case, and, in particular, the review of the work of a custody evaluator appointed by the court. Experts who provide these services need to be highly trained and experienced about how to conduct a child custody evaluation and to efficiently inform the court about issues relevant to divorce, custody, and the best interests of children. The reviewer of the evaluation, or the work product (i.e., report and underlying data collected on the family), may or may not eventually testify in the case. We will argue that all retained experts are consulting to some degree and it is virtually impossible to be a testifying retained expert without consulting with the retaining attorney. This is an important issue since some authorities have proposed that it may be best for testifying experts to limit the amount of consultation they provide (Tippins, 2009; Martindale, 2006a). We argue that these limitations reflect choices made by an attorney for purposes of legal strategy rather than ethical concerns such as a dual role issue, e.g., consulting, reviewing, and testifying.

Roles or Services?

Forensic experts who are involved in custody cases can be differentiated in several keys ways. First, there are evaluators and consultants. Custody evaluators are almost always appointed by the court. They may testify if there is a hearing in the case. A very high percentage of cases settle after the evaluator issues a report. Consultants are always in the role of a retained expert. An attorney may hire the expert to provide consultation services on the case with the understanding that the expert will not become a testifying expert. This role and service is that of a trial consultant and a non-testifying expert-consultant. In other instances, an expert is retained to conduct a work product review. If the expert forms an opinion that the custody evaluation was seriously flawed, then he or she is likely to become a testifying expert-consultant. Some degree of consultation on testimony and trial strategy is likely to occur. This is the role of testifying expert-consultant as a reviewer. Other experts may be asked to provide educational or instructional testimony for the case on research and professional literature that is relevant to the case. Instructional testimony is usually part of the testimony of both the evaluator and reviewer.

The current terms of art for mental health experts in child custody litigation (e.g., evaluator, reviewer, instructor or educator, and consultant) have traditionally been referred to as different "roles" for which the child custody professional community is attempting to define standards (Martindale, 2006a). There has been discussion in attorney trade journal publications on whether an expert should fulfill both reviewer and consultant roles (Tippins, 2009; Martindale, 2006a, 2010). Forensic psychologists have cautioned about a dual role conflict if an expert provides consultation services before conducting a work product review (Heilbrun, 2001). The problem with a role analysis in addressing ethical issues is that roles may be poorly defined and overlapping in their purpose. We propose that the word "services" be used to describe the participation of experts in child custody litigation and that the descriptions of these services include three elements: a description of the service, a description of data or subject matter upon which the task is conducted, and a description of the client for whom the task is performed. For example, what has traditionally been referred to as simply a "child custody evaluation" might be more appropriately identified as "a child custody evaluation of the parties for the court." What has traditionally been referred to as simply a "review" would be "a review of the evaluation report for a party or the court." A "consultant" would more appropriately be described as "a consultant regarding the evaluation/case for a party." Further, we suggest that experts who are providing review testimony or instructional testimony are both consultants in their role as retained experts. They are providing the service of forensic expert testimony, and to varying degrees, case consultation. The evaluator, reviewer, and primarily instructional/educational experts are all providing the forensic service of some degree of instructional testimony for the court. These forensic roles are not distinct.

While we believe it is more helpful to discuss types of forensic services that are provided by evaluators and consultants, it is not possible to completely forsake a role analysis for descriptive purposes. It is important to keep focused on the function of the forensic roles, and not just the label that is attached to the forensic role. There is overlap in ways that are not entirely clear with a superficial examination. For example, the evaluator *reviews* material, documents, records, and reports as part of his or her role and function as an evaluator. Conversely, the reviewer *evaluates* the quality of the evaluator's work product-report and also the professional behavior of the evaluator to determine if the work product quality is discrepant from standard of practice and professional guidelines and standards. In a sense, the evaluator is being evaluated. If, as occasionally will be the case, the evaluator issues a "rebuttal report," in response to an expert reviewer report, then the evaluator is reviewing and evaluating the reviewer's work product. These principal forensic roles in custody disputes can thus be overlapping. The four forensic roles found in custody litigation and their functions are described as follows. The evaluator, reviewer, and instructional testimony experts are testifying roles. The trial consultant is a non-testifying expert to advise the attorney. In addition, the reviewer of an evaluation that is of adequate quality probably will not become a testifying expert and even remain anonymous.

Custody Evaluator

The evaluator is almost always court-appointed after an agreement and stipulation by the parties on the choice of an expert child custody evaluator. If attorneys cannot agree on an evaluator, then the court will designate and appoint one. Typically, several names will be submitted to the court. The evaluator, then, is the court's expert to conduct an objective, impartial, and neutral evaluation that is appropriate to address the issues and questions for the dispute. The order of appointment usually will describe the issues and scope of the evaluation though usually it will be stated generally and there may be a standard form that simply has several boxes checked to denote the issues and scope, for example, parenting time, decision making, and/ or relocation. If there is a very salient issue, such as allegations of domestic violence or substance abuse, then these may be specifically described. Usually, the evaluation will be expected to cover general issues of custody and to be comprehensive. In some jurisdictions (i.e., CA) an order will be issued for a focused-evaluation on one issue and will be very brief in terms of time frame and extent of data collected. The evaluator needs to take care not to exceed the scope of the appointment order, for example, do not investigate relocation if the issue is "not on the table" or contained in the order (see, *In re Marriage of Seagondollar*, 2006). The evaluator can also seek clarification of issues from the attorneys and/or court on what can be investigated or what data can be considered. For example, an evaluator may seek clarification of whether data from a criminal investigation of a parent can be considered in the custody evaluation, if the parent was acquitted. Reviewers usually will examine these issues of scope and consideration of issues and data. Evaluators should always execute a "stipulation" or "statement of understanding" about how forensic and practical matters will be handled in the evaluation so as to make the ground rules and expectations clear. Procedures, fees, and many issues that surround custody evaluations will be described in the stipulation.

If the case goes to trial, it may be expected the evaluator will provide instructional testimony on the research and relevant literature for the court as way to explain the basis or rationale for any opinions and recommendations. The evaluator can also be expected to provide a Case Analysis of the issues in the case in the context of the data and professional literature. This analysis is often accomplished by the use of explanatory concepts (e.g., attachment, parent conflict, parenting style).

The forensic services provided by the evaluator are forensic evaluation and testimony. In some jurisdictions, *ex parté* communication with either attorney during the evaluation or after the release of the custody report may be strictly forbidden by court rules (i.e., CA). In other jurisdictions, consultation with either attorney after the release of the report may occur to facilitate the evaluator's testimony or clarify opinions expressed in the report. If this occurs, the evaluator is also providing a form of forensic consultation service.

Reviewer

The role of reviewer has been described by a limited literature (Gould et al., 2004; Martindale & Gould, 2008; Stahl, 1996; Austin et al., in press;

Martindale, 2010, 2006a; Tippins, 2009). There is agreement that a principal function of the reviewer is to conduct an objective and balanced review of the evaluator's work product-report and to provide candid and fair feedback to the retaining attorney on the strengths as well as any weaknesses of the evaluation. There is consensus in the extant publications that the reviewer will assess the quality of the methodology and procedures in light of the understanding of standard of practice parameters and relevant professional guidelines and standards (i.e., APA, 1994, 2009; AFCC, 2006/2007). There is consensus that the reviewer can and should address the extent that the evaluator's opinions, conclusions, and recommendations offered seem to correspond to the data that were described in the custody report. It appears there would be consensus that the reviewer can appropriately communicate to the retaining attorney on what the correct or more plausible interpretations are concerning issues in the case. Reviewers can address whether the evaluator seemed to adequately and fairly consider all of the relevant alternative hypotheses, or whether there may be confirmatory bias in favor of a preferred hypothesis. It appears there would be agreement among experts that the reviewer could opine to the attorney on what opinions on the ultimate issues seem to fit the case and data as described in the report, but the reviewer would not express ultimate issue opinions in testimony or a report, as we discuss more fully in the following.

There is consensus in the field that the proper reviewer procedure or protocol is to first make it clear to the retaining attorney that the expert-consultant will conduct an objective review of the custody report and formulate opinions about both the strengths and weaknesses of the evaluation (Martindale & Gould, 2008; Austin, Kirkpatrick, & Flens, submitted). A retainer contract should be executed that makes it clear there is no expectation to only focus on deficiencies and that the objective review will be conducted before any consultation services are provided. This is a necessary first step if the reviewer hopes to have any credibility should he or she become a testifying expert (Austin et al., submitted).

The reviewer has a confidential relationship with the retaining attorney in the initial consultation-review stage due to attorney-client privilege (*Hickman v. Taylor*, 1947). Any work product generated by the expert as part of consultation is protected by the attorney-client work product doctrine. If the reviewer communicates to the attorney that there are serious deficiencies based on a reading of the custody report, then it is likely the reviewer will provide testimony as a service. Once the reviewer is identified to the other side and court as a testifying expert the protections of privilege and the work product doctrine are lost and the rules of discovery apply.

After an intense review of the custody report, if the reviewer finds deficiencies, the reviewer will want to examine the evaluator's case file and do further review and analysis. There is a lack of consensus on the issue of whether reviewers can and/or should express opinions on mediate or specific issues based on a review of the evaluator's data. This might be construed as opining about the psychological characteristics of one of the individuals who has not been personally examined and evaluated by the reviewer. This issue of the extent that a mental health professional, who is not an evaluator, can express opinions about persons based on reviewing information is probably much more complicated than is usually appreciated. There is a lack of consistency between ethics and law on this issue as well as ambiguities in the APA Code of Ethics. This is discussed in more detail in the following sections.

The data in the evaluator's case file, including the custody report, are available to the reviewer and thus become the reviewer's data as well. There are numerous advantages to the reviewer and evaluator working from the same dataset. A potential and common problem is poor quality in the evaluator's record in terms of legibility of notes and organization of the file so that it becomes difficult to discern what the data are that served as the basis for the evaluator's opinions (see Austin et al., in press). Generally, the reviewer should not seek or receive new data so as not to appear to slip into the role of evaluator (see Martindale, 2006a; Martindale & Gould, 2008). The same could be said for a reviewer who conducts any interviews with parties or children (AFCC, 2006/2007; Martindale, 2006a). The problem with this is probably not an ethical dual role issue, as the AFCC model standards suggest. Rather, the more pertinent issue is that the reviewer who collects new data is unlikely to have adequate and sufficient data on which to base an opinion (APA, 2002; Rule 9.01(a)). This is similar to the fact that one of the main elements in a review would be to determine if there was an adequate basis for the evaluator's opinions (Martindale, 2006b). The reviewer thus would not be helpful to the court.

The ethical reviewer strives to be helpful to the court and aligned with the data and to provide a balanced analysis of the issues. What is not clear is whether a reviewer should receive and review new data that either stem from new events after the completion of the custody evaluation, or that were data overlooked or not obtained by the evaluator (e.g., school records, DPS records). One viewpoint is that the reviewer role should only encompass a review of the evaluator's methodology and steer clear of any reviewing of material outside of the evaluator's case file (Martindale, 2006b; Martindale & Gould, 2008). The alternative view is that the reviewer should be able to consider, that is, review, "new data" either from new events or obviously pertinent data that were overlooked by the evaluator, in order to be helpful to the court (Austin et al., in press). We also suggest that the court would expect the reviewer expert to opine about new, ostensibly important data. The reviewer could opine about the data in a descriptive way, for example, what the new data are and the implications for the evaluator's opinions. The evaluator, if provided with the data, could opine about the implications for his already expressed opinions. This issue of reviewing new, important data as a reviewer demonstrates the problem of being too focused on roles and prescribed or proscribed behaviors that attach to that role. If the focus is on the forensic service of reviewing pertinent data and documents, either within or outside of the evaluator's case file, then the issue returns to whether there was an adequate basis for the expert's opinion.

Another issue concerning reviewers considering new data is when retained experts listen to courtroom testimony in an extended custody trial. Experts routinely listen to the testimony of other experts in custody trials and even more so in civil litigation. Judges often expect the experts to do so for the purpose of trying to reconcile differences in opinion. Experts on direct and cross-examination will be asked questions about the other expert's testimony. The testimony of the evaluator becomes part of the evaluator's expert output for the court and so it is not problematic for the reviewer to respond to the testimony. It is part of the review process. When the evaluator is asked to respond to the reviewer's rebuttal testimony, then the evaluator is reviewing or "evaluating" the testimony of the reviewer. The evaluator may also have read a report by the reviewer. When a reviewer listens to the testimony of other experts (e.g., therapist, parenting coordinator, school counselor) and fact witnesses, then these are "new data" for the reviewer. Seldom would the evaluator sit in court and listen to other experts (who are not rebuttal experts) or fact witnesses. The evaluator may have interviewed most of such witnesses for the evaluation and report.

This raises the question of whether the reviewer-retained expert may or should opine about the data gleaned from listening to and observing evidence presented in trial. In this instance, admissibility of such testimony would be viewed under the helpfulness standard. The judge and attorneys would be aware that the expert is observing and either had not yet been called as a witness, or could be called as a rebuttal witness and potentially make use of these new, evidentiary data. In a recent case, two of the authors were retained, reviewed experts and listened to testimony in 18 days of trial in a high profile, high conflict case. The witnesses included the parties, a long list of experts who testified on salient issues, teachers, school psychologist, treating psychiatrists, occupational therapists, and a parenting coordinator. Both attorneys and the judge expected the reviewers/experts to respond to questions based on the three weeks of trial.

The issue of whether reviewers should be able to opine on issues based on observing and assimilating testimony of others is not addressed in the literature or professional guidelines. Courtroom-generated data clearly constitute new data. If the reviewer's role is restricted to a methodological critique, then there it might seem there is no reason for the reviewer-retained expert to observe any testimony other than that of the custody evaluator. However, other expert witnesses sometimes reveal data in court that were not obtained by the evaluator or they might dispute the data that were reported by the evaluator.[1] In the aforementioned case, the evaluator destroyed the written notes and created a typed summary of each interview. Professionals who were collaterals in the evaluation testified that the summaries were not correct descriptions of what they had communicated to the evaluator. If the reviewer-retained expert's role is defined that he or she will address mediate issues in the case, based on the evaluator's data, or respond to hypothetical questions about a fact pattern, as permitted in all jurisdictions, then the new data from courtroom observation can be helpful to the court. A key question, then, for the field of child custody and organizations that promulgate professional guidelines is how or should a retained forensic expert be able to address such new data. The court will clearly think this will be helpful and should be permissible. Is this a situation where law and professional ethics are in conflict and the expert witness should refrain from considering the data and therefore choose not to be helpful to the court? The limits and ethics of reviewers' opinion testimony are discussed in future sections.

Instructional Testimony

Instructional (or educational) testimony is defined as expert testimony, including opinion testimony that is explicitly designed to inform and educate the court about specialized, technical, or research-based knowledge as opposed to case-specific testimony. It may involve a summary of research on a particular issue, description of concepts, theory or theoretical frameworks, and forensic models that are relevant to child custody issues. As noted in this article, all testifying experts provide instructional testimony to some degree (Mnookin & Gross, 2003), but they will vary on the emphasis in their testimony and the degree, if any, that the instructional testimony is applied to the facts of the case via use of hypothetical questions.

Some experts provide exclusively instructional or educational testimony. Evaluators enhance case-specific testimony by including a discussion of concepts and research to explain opinions and justify specific recommendations. A reviewer may combine instructional testimony on important issues in the case with case-specific testimony about the forensic quality of the custody evaluation. For example, a reviewer may educate the court about research on overnights in addition to critiquing how the evaluator formulated opinions about this issue based on the data gathered and case circumstances.

When experts combine instructional testimony with their role an overriding goal is to be helpful to the court. Instructional testimony complements and is compatible with the main function of the role of evaluator and reviewer alike. Informing the court about research, theory, and practical considerations surrounding the process of crafting suitable parenting plans is an added benefit to the court. If research hypotheses are relevant and prominent in a case, then the court will benefit from different experts applying the research to the facts of the case, when questions are posed to the expert in hypothetical form.

Mnookin and Gross (2003), in a very scholarly treatment of expert testimony of all sorts, describe instructional testimony and distinguish it from "fact-specific opinion" testimony based on an "assessment" of the data in the case. They indicate that trying to understand the different expert roles "can make the boundaries fuzzy" because all expert testimony is designed to educate the court:

> Experts, to state the obvious, educate—they provide lay people [and judges] with useful information. In court, the only function of an expert witness . . . is to educate, in this very general sense: to supply information that helps the trier of fact make decisions . . . instruction [means providing] general information about some common issue or phenomenon . . . rather than specific information about a particular problem or case . . . Instruction provides background knowledge, but not the case-specific answers. An expert witness who gives purely instructional testimony in a trial can literally repeat the same performance in a different courtroom with a different cast of characters, in another case with a parallel issue with different specific facts. Instructional testimony may lead to an inference that suggests or even requires a specific decision in a case, but it is not itself information about any specific case (pp. 160–161).

Mnookin and Gross (2003) indicate that the boundaries get "fuzzy" between the expert who has conducted the specific assessment in the case and the expert who gives general testimony, then responds to hypothetical questions about a fact pattern, which is allowed under the Federal Rules of Evidence (2008, Rule 702). They cite the well-known example of the expert who is asked about the cause of death of a "hypothetical person" based on a set of presumably hypothetical facts, "but the actual question would incorporate a whole series of *particular* facts that happened to be in evidence in the case at hand, and the expert would provide an opinion assuming these many ostensibly hypothetical facts to be true" (p. 161).

The reviewer must become fully informed about the case-specific information. When there are deficiencies in the evaluation the reviewer is providing assessment of the quality of the assessment of the case-specific data and issues. A reviewer could generally do an adequate assessment of the quality of the methodology in the evaluation without the entire case file, and often the interview notes are not legible. However, in order to adequately determine if the evaluator's opinions correspond to the data, then one obviously needs to review the data. The reviewer will provide case analysis on the issues as part of this assessment in terms of the adequacy of the evaluator's analysis. The reviewer will sometimes provide instructional testimony as part of educating the court on salient issues that the evaluator may have addressed or on research related to these or other issues. The reviewer's testimony thus may be providing *instruction* and also addressing case-specific information that was part of the evaluation. As Mnookin and Gross (2003) point out, "Whatever the dividing line between instruction and assessment, most experts—and certainly most expert witnesses—go back and forth across it and provide both types of information" (p. 161). This statement reflects our position on why it is more helpful to discuss forensic services and the purpose of the service for the court and retaining attorney rather than saying the service is specific to a forensic role.

When experts are dedicated, instructional testimony experts they can be described as providing "case blind didactic testimony" (Martindale & Gould, 2008):

> A case-blind educator provides information concerning some well-researched dynamic and leaves it to the court to decide how (if at all) the dynamic that has been explained is applicable to the issues in dispute. The concept is not a new one; other writers (for example, Vidmar and Schuller, 1989) have used the term "social framework testimony." Our preference for the term "case-blind didactic testimony" lies in the fact that the words "case-blind" emphasize the importance of diligently maintaining constructive ignorance of the facts of the case (p. 536).

Martindale and Gould put forth an interesting concept, but this practice is rare and probably limited to those situations where a retaining attorney believes the court needs to be educated on the research or a particular concept, or perhaps a forensic model for evaluators. When the expert is "blind" to the facts, then the expectation would be that the testifying expert's credibility would be enhanced. If, however, a hypothetical question and fact pattern would be posed, then that strategic advantage might be lost. It is much more common for the testifying expert to be aware of the facts of the case when general testimony is provided. Usually, the expert will be asked to apply the research to a hypothetical fact pattern.

Non-Testifying Consultant

The final forensic role in child custody litigation is that of the expert who strictly offers consultation service for the retaining attorney as a non-testifying consultant. The range of services include educating the attorney and her client about the professional literature on important issues; helping with trial strategy and with the development a "theory for the case" for litigation; and drafting questions for direct and cross-examination of witnesses. The consultant often would sit near the attorney during trial to provide advice. The work product produced by the non-testifying consultant would be covered by attorney-client work product privilege and could not be discovered by the other attorney. The consultant usually would also meet with the attorney's client and could gather information from the client for the purpose of trial preparation.

As discussed in the following, there are different viewpoints in the field on whether or to what extent a testifying expert should provide consultation services to the retaining attorney. The pros and cons will be discussed. When the testifying expert, a reviewer, also provides consultation, then a draw-back from a legal strategy point of view, for example, the retaining attorney's perspective, is that the work product would be discoverable or available to the other side (Tippins, 2009).

Case Analysis as Part of Expert Opinions and Testimony

We define case analysis as the description, consideration, and analysis of the salient case issues, psycho-legal questions, and mediate and ultimate issues in the context of the case. It often involves integrating relevant research, conceptual frameworks, and practical considerations with the issues of the case. Case analysis involves either an implicit or explicit analytical process in every custody evaluation and we recommend it should be an explicit component in the work product review as well. Part of what the reviewer is assessing is the quality of the evaluator's case analysis. If the evaluator used a concept or series of concepts or drew upon the research literature to frame the issues and data for the court and to offer explanations for the opinions, then the reviewer will assess how the "social framework" was constructed and applied, as well as if it was a relevant and useful framework. A framework can be misleading or based on a weak or inconsistent research literature. For example, an evaluator might use Parental Alienation Syndrome to describe a mother's attempts to limit the father's involvement or to want to set conditions for parenting time. The reviewer might suggest, however, that a history of intimate partner violence, as contained in the evaluator's investigation, provided rational reasons for the mother's actions and a better framework and concept would have been to view the mother as a "protective gatekeeper" (Austin & Drozd, 2006; Austin, Flens, & Kirkpatrick, 2010). All of the testifying forensic roles usually include case analysis and educative testimony to some degree. Case analysis is a central forensic service that is integrated into the roles of evaluator and reviewer in their reports and testimony.

Combining Forensic Expert Services

A limited literature has addressed whether forensic experts can ethically combine the forensic roles of case consultation and giving expert testimony. The main concern is whether the process and sequence of providing consultation services somehow creates bias or other distortions into the expert's opinion (Heilbrun, 2001). It seems mandatory that a reviewer should first conduct an objective review before agreeing to engage in case consultation, for example, advising about case issues and strategy, and preparing questions for expert examination (Martindale & Gould, 2008; Heilbrun, 2001). In a role analysis, this issue would be framed as the advisability of operating in a "hybrid role" that combines the functions of reviewing work product, consultation, testimony, and providing instructional testimony. We believe this issue is better described as an expert combining forensic services and trying to do so in an ethical manner as prescribed by the APA code of ethics (APA, 2002, Rule 9.01) so the expert is required to base opinions on necessary and sufficient information.

Forensic experts always combine services as described previously. When the reviewer or evaluator includes case analysis and instructional testimony there is no conflict in function. The experts are trying to be helpful to the court. Conflicts potentially arise when the retained expert provides more than one forensic service and there is reason to believe that something has compromised or impaired the expert's objectivity. Our view is that some degree of consultation is necessary to facilitate the efficient production of the expert's testimony and opinions. The principle of the retained expert striving to be helpful to the court by remaining true to the data is discussed in the following sections. We suggest that consultation with the retaining attorney is necessary to be most helpful to the court though there could be a debate about what types of consultation are advisable for the reviewer. We suggest the reviewer should assist the attorney in the preparation of questions for his or her direct examination in order to be effective and helpful to the court.

Two authorities, publishing in attorney trade journals, have recommended that it would be best, or ideal, if the reviewer-testifying and forensic consultation roles are bifurcated and not mixed in these functions (Tippins, 2009; Martindale, 2006a, 2010). Both Tippins and Martindale emphasize the need for the proper sequence for the reviewer to first conduct an objective review before considering an offer to provide consultation services and that this approach should be in a retainer contract (Martindale, 2010). Neither authority seems to feel there is anything inherently unethical about providing both services to the attorney, even though it might be construed as a "dual role" situation for the expert. Both authorities point out that the issue of combining roles (e.g., services) relate to the perception of credibility and the testifying reviewer-consultant being subject to discovery. Therefore, the main drawback with combining services would be one of legal strategy and effectiveness of the expert witness. Both authorities indicate the ethical reviewer can be helpful to the court and potentially effective if there is balanced analysis and allegiance with the data rather than assuming the attorney's advocacy position. Both authorities also recommend that the best approach is to bifurcate the roles so there is a testifying reviewer-expert who does not consult and a consulting expert who does not testify. The two experts, then, would be part of the attorney's "litigation team" (Tippins, 2009). Our position is that it is unrealistic to believe the testifying reviewer would not provide some degree of consultation to enhance the efficacy of her testimony, even though it might be that little or no written work product would be produced. Tippins (2009) acknowledges that most clients cannot afford to hire two experts. Martindale (2010) also points out while retained experts-reviewers can conduct objective reviews and that stay aligned and loyal to the data, the reviewer must be able to resist the built-in pressure to try to please the person who is paying for the services which Martindale describes as "retention bias."

Retained, testifying experts are often not perceived as objective in the same way as the court's appointed neutral expert in the sense that the court expects the expert's testimony will generally be supportive of retaining attorney's legal position. However, for the ethical reviewer, it should be the case that he or she is testifying because their objective view of the data is consistent with the position of the attorney who offers them as an expert. This is part of the need of the expert to be true to the sworn oath for testimony. Retained experts are supposed to give an objective and fair analysis of the data in the evaluator's file, the research literature, and an accurate application to the issues in the case. It is up to the court to decide if the retaining expert's testimony is reasonably objective, accurate, and credible despite the fact that the retained, testifying expert is being retained, presented by, and paid by the retaining attorney.

The cross-examining attorney will try to portray the retained expert as a "hired gun," even if steps are taken for the expert not to provide any consultation. Providing consultation services in addition to testimony has the added drawback that the testimony may be perceived as less credible because the expert may be perceived by the court as too aligned with the position of one side. But this is not always the case, particularly when experts remain objective and true to the data of the evaluation. The court often is an astute discerner of competent, balanced, and accurate testimony. The data are what they are, so to speak, and the issues are what they are. The court will usually know which expert "got it right" in the description and analysis of the data. The downside to the expert combining forensic services of testimony and consultation, then, is one of effectiveness and perceived credibility. It is not unethical to do so according to any professional guidelines or standards. When other types of professionals provide forensic testimony (e.g., medical malpractice), it is often the case that consultation is combined with testimony. The expert may even start out strictly as a consultant and then it is decided he will provide testimony.

Our experience is that testifying reviewers, who also provide consultation, can be very effective witnesses and perceived by the court as credible depending on their qualifications, reputation, and the balance and accuracy in their testimony. While the retaining attorney may cringe at the thought of his consulting expert's work product being disclosed (e.g., questions prepared for direct or cross-examination), the ethical retained expert would not despair because the focus would be on being true to the data and issues. The reviewer who helps the attorney prepare questions for his own testimony, or that of others, is helping to facilitate the discovery of relevant and important evidence for the court. The reviewer-consultant role and function thus can be viewed as being helpful to the retaining attorney and court. It would appear when the retained expert first conducts the objective review before moving into providing complementary consulting services, then this would be acceptable practice. When the expert starts off with consulting and then moves toward reviewing and testifying, then this would be an unacceptable sequence of forensic services if the reviewer's objectivity is lost. We feel if there was a bright line rule that reviewers could not also consult with the retaining attorney, then there would be rare for attorneys to retain reviewers.

Some commentators view combining of testimony and consultation as a dual role issue. It would seem Heilbrun (2001) takes this position only if consultation services, or consulting role, precedes the objective work product review. The AFCC Model Standards (Rule 8.5) discusses a dual role problem for reviewers (ironically, titled "Role Delineation in Consulting") only in regard to reviewers needing to avoid having a relationship with either party in the litigation in light of the professional relationship with the retaining attorney. Combining work product review, expert testimony, and consultation for the same retaining attorney is not a multiple role. They are separate services provided to the same person and in the same general consulting role with the attorney.

This situation, in our opinion, would not fall within the APA standard involving multiple relationships. The APA Code addresses the issue of multiple relationships in terms of the likelihood of impairing objectivity, effectiveness, or exploiting others: "A psychologist refrains from entering a multiple relationship if the multiple relationship could reasonably be expected to impair the psychologist's objectivity, competence, or effectiveness in performing his or her functions as a psychologist, or otherwise risks exploitation or harm to the person with whom the professional exists. Multiple relationships that would not reasonably be expected to cause impairment or risk of exploitation or harm are not unethical" (APA, 2002, Rule 3.05(a), p. 1065). One could argue that combining testifying and consulting would inherently impede objectivity, but authorities have written eloquently how retained experts routinely face and can overcome this challenge by being true to the data and issues and providing balanced reasoning and analysis for the courts, as is common practice in civil litigation (Shuman & Greenberg, 2003). Forensic psychologists routinely work within this context of tension between law and professional ethics and follow the dictum of the forensic Specialty Guidelines to strive for objectivity in analysis and opinions no matter who has requested the forensic services (Committee on Ethical Guidelines for Forensic Psychologists, 1991). The provision in the APA Code about the risk of exploiting the person in the professional relationship is a realistic concern, but it should be manageable for the ethical expert.

EXPERT TESTIMONY AS SOCIAL INFLUENCE

All forensic testifying experts are engaging in a process of social influence and persuasion (Shuman & Greenberg, 2003). They are communicating with the court and trying to influence the opinion of the decision maker on a variety of mediate and ultimate issues in the case. The expert wants the court to view him or her as knowledgeable, comprehensive, and insightful on issues that need to be addressed. The expert wants the court to believe that he or she figured out the main issues and basically "got it right" on the ultimate issues. In the case of custody disputes this process of social influence takes the form of describing the issues in the case, presenting data on the results of investigation of the parties and children, and providing very specific recommendations on a parenting plan the court should address. In most jurisdictions, the judge presiding over a child custody dispute expects evaluators to formulate and express ultimate issue opinions and recommendations. Experienced evaluators are accustomed to judges generally following their recommendations thus completing the process of social influence.

Experts, evaluators and reviewers, want to be helpful to the court, but they also want to be effective. Both experts may be offering instructional testimony on issues and the professional literature. The evaluator offers opinions on a best interest parenting plan and gives testimony on the rationale for the recommended plan for parenting time and how decision making should be shared. The reviewer's communication and attempt at social influence with the court come in the form of opinions on the quality of evaluation, including whether the data support the evaluator's ultimate issue opinions. The reviewer will communicate if the methodology and overall quality of the evaluation meets minimum standards in terms of methodology and analysis. It is not often that the court will disregard completely the forensic findings and opinions, but this does happen when there is a very poor evaluation and the reviewer provides influential testimony. The reviewer provides an important checks and balances function for the court.

HELPFULNESS IN THE ROLE AND EVALUATOR AND REVIEWER

The main purpose of expert testimony is to be helpful to the court. This is true for the role of the testifying court evaluator and all testifying retained experts. Whether the purpose of the retained expert is to provide rebuttal testimony to the evaluator's testimony and/or give general, instructional testimony, the overriding principle to guide the evaluator should be to try to be helpful to the court. This is accomplished by every expert attempting to be true to the data and issues, and to present a balanced analysis for the court. Only in this way will the court view the expert as credible. Only by attempting to provide a balanced analysis that treats the data and issues with objectivity will the expert be effective and persuasive. The reviewer needs to solve the puzzle of how to be effective and persuasive by appearing to be aligned with the data and not the advocacy of the retaining attorney (Tippins, 2009). Everyone is aware that the retaining attorney has hired the expert to provide forensic services (as opposed to being appointed by the court) and expects the reviewer's testimony will be favorable to her position and client so it is a challenge for the retained expert to achieve credibility in the eyes of the court. This is a commonplace legal context for the forensic mental health expert in civil litigation.

An "integrated approach" to providing ethical testimony in the role of the retained expert is presented by Shuman and Greenberg (2003). It will be easier for the retained expert who only provides general, educational testimony, for example, describing the research and professional literature, to be perceived as credible compared to the reviewer. For example, if the expert appears to testify about the issue and research on overnight parenting time for very young children and does not critique how the evaluator handled this position, then the issue of alignment probably becomes a non-issue. Our ethics require us to be objective in our interpretation of data and analysis. This point can be made by the reviewer in testimony and a forensic report which may serve to bolster credibility. The Specialty Guidelines (Committee on Ethical Guidelines for Forensic Psychologists, 1991) describes the need for objectivity no matter who has requested the forensic services:

> In providing forensic psychological services, forensic psychologists take special care to avoid undue influence upon their methods, procedures, and products, such as might emanate from the party to a legal proceeding by financial compensation or other gains. As an expert conducting an evaluation, treatment, consultation, or scholarly/empirical investigation, the forensic psychologist maintains professional integrity by examining the issue at hand from all reasonable perspectives, actively seeking information that will differentially test plausible rival hypotheses (p. 341).

The controlling federal case on admissibility for expert testimony (*Daubert v. Merrell Dow Pharmaceuticals, Inc.*, 1993) described the main rule on expert testimony in the Federal Rules of Evidence (Rule 702) as the helpfulness standard (*Daubert*, p. 2796). Most states pattern their rules of evidence after the federal rules. On this issue, then, the law and professional ethics converge. If the court believes the reviewer, or any retained expert, is balanced, objective, and accurate in his or her opinions, then credibility will be established.

The federal standard on admitting and weighting expert testimony (*Daubert*, 1993; FRE, 2008) is defined in terms of adequacy of the data, reliable procedures or methods, and correct application of principles and methods. It would seem that this would be consistent with a practical application of gatekeeping by family law judges. Courts want to determine if the evaluator collected the necessary types of data from multiple sources and using multiple methods; if the analysis was cogent, appeared balanced, and offered without bias; and if the salient questions were reasonably addressed. Reviewers would be expected to apply the same questions in the work product review.

When, or if, the court examines the admissibility of expert testimony by a reviewer it would not be on criteria of reliability or the typical *Daubert* criteria (1993) because there has not been an evaluation. The concept of reliability would not be relevant. Testimony that is strictly a review of methodology and assessment of the quality of the evaluation will be gauged in terms of the general interpretation of helpfulness. If the reviewer provides instructional testimony on research and professional consensus of opinion on an issue (e.g., child alienation), then this could be challenged on the grounds of relevance and validity of the research cited.

SCIENTIFICALLY GROUNDED EXPERT TESTIMONY AND ADMISSIBILITY

Expert testimony by evaluators is expected to be scientifically-grounded to some degree (Gould, 2006; Gould & Martindale, 2007) which is not say that custody evaluations do not depend on clinical-forensic skill and experience. Evaluators exercise discretionary judgment on what questions to ask and data to collect and utilize clinical judgment to form hypotheses that need to be investigated. Psychologist child custody evaluators (and reviewers) need to be mindful of their "Code of Conduct" that states as a standard "Psychologists' work is based upon established scientific and professional knowledge of the discipline" (APA, 2002, Rule 2.04, p. 1064).

There clearly is an art as well as a science dimension to forensic custody evaluation. The evaluator needs to have knowledge that is grounded in the scientific research literature in psychology and related fields. The evaluator needs to employ reliable and valid procedures for collecting data. Interviews and observations of parents and children, and interviews with third parties, are the main source of direct data for the evaluator. These are qualitative, descriptive data not derived from scientific procedures. The overall evaluation protocol, however, needs to be systematic, comprehensive, and use multiple methods and multiple sources of information so that it is likely to produce the necessary and sufficient data to answer the required questions. Psychological testing will be the most scientific data in an evaluation. The evaluator needs to be mindful not to use blatantly unreliable procedures and base decisions in whole or part on those unreliable procedures.

For example, if an evaluator used human figure drawings and relied upon the drawings to draw conclusions about a child or parent, then there would be a risk of those opinions being disregarded by the court. When it is competently designed and implemented, the overall package of the custody evaluation will be seen by the court as sufficiently reliable and robust in order to be admitted into evidence and considered. How scientific a custody report is will vary with the expertise and approach of the evaluator. Courts will at least view custody evaluations, reports, and testimony as potentially useful "specialized knowledge." Shuman and Sales (1998) suggested that custody evaluation expert testimony would fall in the category of "clinical opinion testimony" and, thus, would not need to be held to a standard of being sufficiently scientifically grounded, or based upon reliable and valid scientific methodology and knowledge.

The standard or degree of rigor that courts use to assess the admissibility of expert child custody work product and testimony is important for both the evaluator and reviewer to know. The evaluator needs to plan and gauge his or her approach and choice of methodology on an understanding of this issue if he or she wants to be effective and persuasive as an expert. The reviewer similarly needs to cognizant of this issue and the standard being employed by the court as the regulator of expert testimony in order to effectively communicate with the court about the quality of the evaluator's work product. Generally, issues of admissibility and weight assigned to expert opinion testimony need to have a reliable and valid basis. The reviewer can assist the court in this assessment of the evaluator's work product.

In FRE (2008), Rule 702 states:

"If scientific, technical, or other specialized knowledge will assist the trier of fact to understand the evidence or to determine a fact in issue, a witness qualified as an expert by knowledge, skill, experience, training, or education, may testify thereto in the form of an opinion or otherwise, if (1) the testimony is based upon sufficient facts or data, (2) the testimony is the product of reliable principles and methods, and (3) the witness has applied the principles and methods reliably to the facts of the case" (p. 127).

The three tenets in this core rule govern issues of admissibility and/or giving weight to expert testimony. They alert the evaluator and guide the reviewer in the assessment of the evaluator's work product. The custody evaluation with poor methodology that is conducted by a qualified evaluator is unlikely to be excluded by the court, but it may be given little or no weight if the court finds the reviewer's testimony convincing.

CONFIRMATORY BIAS AND THE ETHICAL EXPERT

In a survey of judges and attorneys, Bow and Quinnell (2004) reported that the issue that most concerned the legal professions in custody evaluation was the need for objectivity by the court evaluator. It is not uncommon for experienced Reviewers to encounter work products where there appears to be bias operating in terms of data interpretation and opinions. Evaluators are the court's expert and they are charged with an obligation to conduct a neutral and objective evaluation. Bias may arise from personal experience with a litigant during the evaluation; from selectively considering preferred hypotheses or social frameworks; from misguided interpretations of a primary explanatory concept; or from a selective view of empirical generalizations from the research literature.

Custody litigants are an extreme group in a number of ways. First, statistically, most child custody cases settle without a court hearing, estimated to be about 90% of all cases (e.g., Melton et al., 2007). Of the cases that do not settle, only in a small percentage of these lead to a CCE. Thus, it is this small group that gets funneled toward an evaluator. Second, custody litigants report a high frequency of intimate partner violence (Newmark, Harrell, & Salem, 1995) and this can elicit negative feelings by an evaluator; this can be called, "parent conduct bias." Third, it is accepted by forensic evaluators that there will be a high percentage of difficult personalities or even parties with personality disorders within this population. For these reasons, the evaluator needs to guard for negative reactions (Martindale & Gould, 2007) or even counter-transference (Pickar, 2007). Evaluators, not infrequently, will find these folks to be not very likeable. The "likeability bias," either being "turned-off" by the actions and/or personality of an offensive litigant or being impressed by positive qualities and/or charm of a litigant, is not uncommon. Evaluators need to be very vigilant and on guard for this affective bias. A less likeable parent may be the more effective parent who does a better job in managing the needs of the child. Reviewers sometimes find, unfortunately it seems, the evaluator simply liked one parent more than the other and this seems to account for the recommendations to the court.

Reviewers can provide a useful service to the court and the litigation by monitoring the evaluator's report for potential bias. In this sense, Reviewers are a type of conscience for the profession and watchdog for the court. Perhaps the most common error and source of bias is that of not considering, in an open and fair way, all of the relevant, alternative rival hypotheses on each important issue. The concept of confirmatory bias was borrowed from cognitive psychology and introduced to the field of child custody (Martindale, 2005). Due to review work that is being provided across the United States, it is not unusual for judges and attorneys to express familiarity with the concept and issue of confirmatory bias. This term refers to the natural human cognitive process to interpret and filter information in way that favors a preferred hypothesis. When this process is operating, confirmatory information is noted and weighted, while disconfirming data are discounted, ignored, or given little weight. It is assumed this is an unintentional or unconscious process. When it appears the evaluator is intentionally ignoring information, then the sister concept of confirmatory distortion (Martindale, 2005) applies and can be used to describe this phenomenon to the court. For example, in a recent case, the evaluator testified that psychological testing was the least important data source in the evaluation. As a result, extreme psychological testing profiles were given little weight on the implications for parenting and co-parenting. This was the evaluator's opinion, even though there were corroborating data from other sources and procedures that could have been predicted from the actual psychological testing data. In another case, the evaluator described how he tried to talk a mother out of wanting to relocate with her young child from one state to another, so there was a preconception or negative mindset about relocation. When there is clear and potent confirmatory bias or confirmatory distortion operating, the quality of the work product will be poor and there will probably be a fatal flaw in terms of the custody evaluation's helpfulness to the court. Confirmatory bias is operating when the evaluator clearly is not gathering or interpreting data in a balanced and even-handed way.

Using preferred concepts and not relying on the research literature can also produce a confirmatory or distorted cognitive process. For example, it is not unusual to concepts such as primary caregiver, primary attachment figure, parental alienation, or "batterer" to be a primary force in data interpretation and formulating opinions. Concepts and research can be extremely helpful in framing issues for the court, educating the court, and interpreting the data if they do not interfere with fair consideration of alternative hypotheses. Concepts help the evaluator interpret and explain data. They assist the reviewer in critiquing the evaluator and in providing instructional testimony, but "concept-generated confirmatory bias" can occur for either the evaluator or reviewer. Substantive issues, and the evaluator's personal and professional opinion about that issue, can also create a cognitive lens to drive a one-sided analysis. Evaluator's opinions about relocation, which can be based on scientific research, can result in a distorted analysis of the issue. Our experience as evaluators suggests an anti-relocation basis is widespread even though very few states have a legal presumption for relocation by the children with a custodial parent (Atkinson, 2010). This type of "issue-generated confirmatory bias" (Bala, 2004) is also encountered when other substantive issues are salient and the focus of the case. In addition, recent advances in the field on intimate partner violence (IPV) have encouraged evaluators and other professionals to approach this issue with an open mind and an understanding that there are many behavioral variations when IPV has occurred in relationship (Kelly & Johnson, 2008; Ver Steegh, 2005). Some evaluators still follow the view that all IPV represents "battering" in a stereotyped approach to the issue.

Our experience is that testimony by reviewers can also come across as biased just as evaluator's are frequently perceived as biased. It is understandable when the reviewer appears to be marching to the beat of the retaining attorney. Reviewers who are not following their ethical guidelines of strict adherence to objectivity and following the data (Committee on Ethical Guidelines for Forensic Psychologists, 1991) can thus play into the preconception of the defensive evaluator or others in the case that the reviewer is nothing more than a "hired gun." And, well, he or she may be, if the reviewer is caught up in his or her own bias and distorting data interpretation from the evaluator's file with the goal of supporting the advocacy position of the attorney rather than advocating for the data (Tippins, 2009).

ETHICAL REVIEW WORK: HIRED GUN OR FORENSIC QUALITY CONTROL?

Evaluators often look upon Reviewers as a "hired gun" or as someone who is tainted and inherently biased in favor of the retaining attorney. The retained expert-reviewer may be seen as a mercenary. The other attorney will usually try to portray the retained expert-reviewer in this way. However, as noted previously, an evaluator who is reviewed may not see or ever even know about a reviewer who found the work product to be satisfactory, gave the retaining attorney candid feedback that the evaluation was acceptable on methodology, and opined that the evaluator seemed to get it right for the court on the ultimate issues. The ethical reviewer who describes the strengths as well as weaknesses for the retaining attorney may instead be asked to continue as a consultant, or be discharged from further service. We find that attorneys often are astute consumers of mental health work products. They generally identify situations where the evaluation is inadequate, or that "I know bias when I see it." Thus, the frequency of evaluations/reports that are of excellent quality rarely may be identified for a review. The astute referring/retaining attorney presumably also will know an accurate and well-balanced report/evaluation when he or she sees it.

Because a review of the quality of the evaluator's work product is not a dichotomous assessment, a review typically finds some weaknesses in method and procedure, but also strengths. It also may be the case that while the evaluation contained questionable use of procedures, data gathering, or formulation of opinions, the reviewer concluded that the evaluator "basically got it right for the court" on the bottom line of the recommended parenting plan. For example, the evaluator may have misinterpreted the psychological testing data, but it appears the necessary and sufficient data were competently collected so that the ultimate issue recommendations seemed to be adequately supported. The ethical reviewer will not suggest that the attorney rush through a small opening created by one methodological flaw to try to discredit the entire report. Doing so would be to waste the court's time on irrelevant detail.

The ethical responsibility of the reviewer is to be true to the data that are collected by the evaluator and to objectively consider all plausible interpretations of the data. Our ethical responsibility as reviewers is the same as the evaluator; to "get it right" for the Court with an eye towards the Court's role to make a determination on the best interests of the child. The ethical analysis and testimony of the reviewer requires the same type of stringent adherence to objectivity and to be scientifically-grounded in the analysis just as the evaluator.

Ethical reviewers and consultants cannot remove themselves from their scientific training to pursue the "truth." By being truthful in their testimony and following the data, the reviewer as a testimonial expert can be helpful to the court and the legal process and therefore indirectly be helpful to the children and parties. Perhaps the strongest argument that can be made that for ethical reviewer testimony is the obvious point that the expert is under oath to tell the truth. The reviewer cannot escape the adversarial context of litigation which is designed to help the court uncover the truth and the best interests of the children by way of hearing advocacy from two competing advocates. The testimonial expert, evaluator or reviewer, does not get to ask the questions. By testifying in a truthful and balanced manner on the work product quality and data in the case file, it is inevitable that the attorney who is performing either direct or cross-examination will want to highlight the strengths of his or her case. Questions the expert wants to be asked may not be posed, but there is high probability they will be. After all, when the expert is cross-examined it is the attorney's turn to "testify" by asking leading questions and uncovering every relevant issue. What the expert wants to communicate should not be constrained too much if both attorneys are doing their job well. Plus, some judges are disposed to grant experts fairly wide latitude in answering questions. We have found that the best outcome in reviewer testimony is when the judge "psychologically hires" the reviewer's opinion and asks questions of the reviewer from the bench.

While the ethical duty of the retained, testifying expert is to be true to the data and issues and to be helpful to the court, the expert would not be testifying if the thrust of the testimony was not going to be helpful to the retaining attorney and his or her client, for example, one of the litigants. For this reason, the other attorney on cross-examination will try to paint the reviewer as a "hired gun" and will ask how much money the expert is receiving for his services. In very complicated cases with large case files, the fees can be quite impressive so the other attorney will argue there is a correlation between the size of the fees and how favorable the testimony is for the other side. Martindale (2010) suggests there can be "retention bias" where the expert may feel "subtle pressure to please those who have paid for our services" (p. 6). He adds, "It becomes the obligation of retained testifying experts and the attorneys who retain them to take reasonable steps to reduce the impact of retention bias." The way to overcome unintentional pressure to please would seem for the retained, testifying expert to stay mindful of the issues, the obligation to be helpful to the court, and to be true to the data in the case file and evidence presented, if the reviewer observes testimony. Tippins (2009) points out the credibility of the testifying, retained expert will be enhanced if the expert is perceived as advocating for the data and not for the litigation position. Judges are looking for accurate testimony regardless of the forensic role of the expert. The passage from the Specialty Guidelines (Committee on Ethical Guidelines for Forensic Psychologists, 1991), as quoted previously, needs to be kept in mind as an ethical mantra. This standard on the evaluator's neutrality and close adherence to the case data should be part of a reviewer's professional policy and should be described in the retainer contract with the attorney.

Martindale (2006a) points out that there are different types of "hired guns" in the role of retained expert, or ethical and unethical review testimony:

> There is an important distinction between principled hired guns and unprincipled hired guns. Unprincipled hired guns will testify to any opinion that someone pays them to testify to, will cite research that they know to be flawed, and will be unconcerned that they are misleading judges. Principled hired guns are knowledgeable and familiar with applicable research; able to discern the difference between sound methodology and flawed methodology; able to interpret test data without computer-generated interpretive reports; and, have formulated opinions on various issues based upon their studies. Inevitably, there will be times when an opinion held by the practitioner is precisely the opinion that a particular attorney wants a judge to hear. When the principled expert is paid to come to court and explain that opinion to the judge, the expert is being paid for time expended and nothing more. The principled retained expert takes seriously the most basic obligation of an expert witness—the obligation to assist the trier of fact (p. 4).

The tension between the various views of retained experts-reviewers as hired guns—can be diffused if the reviewer remains mindful of the helpfulness principle. The attitude of the judge towards the rebuttal expert, after all, is more important than the perceptions or assumptions of the evaluator. Martindale (2006b) again describes how the issue of helpfulness underlies ethical reviewer testimony and serves to enhance the expert's credibility:

> Testimony by reviewing experts is most effective when they are perceived by the court as practitioners with a genuine interest in educating judges concerning good methodology, flawed methodology, and the ways in which methodological errors can lead evaluators to make misguided recommendations. If experts who are endeavoring to educate judges regarding methodological flaws in evaluations are asked on cross-examination whether they have met with or discussed the case with any of the interested parties, the usefulness of the experts' testimony is dependent upon their responses. Just as evaluators must employ sound methodology or face the consequences of not having done so when they

encounter a skilled cross-examining attorney, so too must Reviewers employ sound methodology or face well-deserved jabs at their credibility during cross-examination. Experts who have had contact with litigants, family members, or allies are likely to be perceived as less objective, as less devoted to sound methodology, and, therefore, as less credible (p. 4).

OPINIONS REVIEWERS CAN OR SHOULD OFFER

Rules of evidence (FRE, 2008, Rule 702) permit experts to offer opinions on mediate or ultimate issues except for the question of mental status at the time of offense for criminal defendants (i.e., *mens rea*). There is controversy in the field of child custody on whether evaluator experts should address the ultimate issue (Tippins & Wittmann, 2005; Bala, 2005), but there appears to be a consensus that judges expect the court's expert will make specific recommendations on parenting time, decision making, and other salient issues (Stahl, 2005; Gould & Martindale, 2005; Martin, 2005).

While there are voices in the field that question how scientifically-grounded custody evaluators can be (Emery et al., 2005), it is clear that federal and most state rules of evidence direct the court to use the lens of a scientific or reliable foundation for testimony. The methods of the expert need to rely on general acceptance, reliability, and/or a systematic approach to the issue before the court so the opinions are more likely to be accurate and/or reliable. The FRE states experts "may testify . . . if (1) the testimony is based on sufficient facts or data, (2) the testimony is the product of reliable principles and methods, and (3) the witness has applied the principles and methods reliably to the facts of the case" (p. 126). The FRE and comparable state rules do not differentiate between court-appointed and retained experts and the expectation in the drafting of the rules was probably that most often the experts would be retained experts in either civil litigation or criminal proceedings. There are few constraints on what opinions the expert can express as long as the criteria of relevance, reliability, and helpfulness are met. There is no distinction between experts who have conducted a case-specific assessment vs. instructional expert testimony (i.e., see Mnookin & Gross, 2003 discussed previously). However, as we will see, the discipline of psychology and its ethics code asserts this distinction is very important. It is this tension in the ethics code that poses difficulties and limitations for the opinions the reviewer can or should express.

While the literature on the reviewer role and services is limited and guidelines not yet developed, there appears to be disagreement on what opinions reviewers can or should offer in a custody case. We feel the field of child custody evaluation and the discipline of forensic psychology needs to closely examine this issue. The issue concerns to what extent the retained expert, who has not performed a direct assessment, can opine on the issues directly in dispute in the case and/or offer interpretations and opinions concerning the case-specific data. Specifically, if the reviewer has closely examined the custody report and the entire case file, should the reviewer be limited to opining only on the quality of the evaluator's methodology? That would seem to be only partially helpful to the court. Can the reviewer opine if the evaluator's opinions correspond to the underlying data, or in other words, if the evaluator correctly interpreted the data? It appears the emerging literature from noted experts in the field agree the reviewer should be able to opine about the evaluator's methodology and if the data support the proffered opinions (Martindale, 2010; Martindale & Gould, 2008). However, these experts and pioneers in the field seem to hold the position that the reviewer ought not to offer opinions on substantive issues in the case based on the data reviewed and certainly should not opine about the psychological characteristics of the individuals who have not been personally examined.

The legal parameters vary substantially between jurisdictions on whether a reviewer should be able to opine based only on a review of records, documents, and so forth, and without a direct assessment of an individual. For example, in North Carolina, case law specifically holds that an expert can opine about an individual based on a sufficient review of records and written information and without having directly evaluated the individual in question (*State of North Carolina v. Daniels*, 1994). However, in many other jurisdictions the mental health expert needs to personally examine the person in order to give expert testimony about a mental condition or diagnosis (*Holloway v. State*, 1981; *People v. Wilson*, 1987). The psychological or psychiatric interview has long been viewed as an integral part, and possibly necessary component, before an expert offers an opinion about a clinical diagnosis (*Rollerson v. United States*, 1964).

The issue here is multifaceted. It concerns whether the expert who has not personally evaluated a party or child can or should offer an opinion about personal or psychological characteristics, offer a diagnosis, or address the ultimate issues for the court. It is well established that experts can give opinions in response to questions about hypothetical issues and facts if the facts have been admitted into evidence or are expected to be placed into evidence. The U.S. Supreme Court ruled in *Barefoot v. Estelle* (1983), a fairly famous death penalty case:

> Jury should not be barred from hearing views of the state's psychiatrists along with opposing views of the defendant's doctors as to defendant's dangerousness ... expert opinions, whether in form of opinion based on hypothetical questions or otherwise, ought in general to be deduced from facts that are not disputed, or from facts given in evidence, but may be founded upon statement of facts proved in the case rather than upon personal knowledge, and even in cases involving death penalty there is no constitutional barrier to applying ordinary rules of evidence governing use of expert testimony including use of hypothetical questions ... (p. 463).

Thus, experts, who have not performed a direct assessment, but are fully informed about the facts in the case (and a custody evaluator's entire file) may opine in response to hypothetical questions about fact patterns that essentially refer to the real facts or data in the case. Responding to questions in hypothetical form thus creates an ethical safe haven and is permitted under FRE 702, *Barefoot v. Estelle 1983*, and most state case law. In this context, the APA Code of Conduct (2002) needs to be closely examined to give guidance to reviewers as to what types of opinions they should express. It should be noted that the field of psychology seems to impose much more stringent standards on its members on this issue than any other profession. In addition, we are unaware of any national organization guidelines on forensic practice for any other mental health profession, e.g., licensed professional counselors or social workers.

This issue of the limits of expert opinion, where there has not been a personal assessment, is one where what may be permitted legally by rules of evidence, case law, and trial courts may be discrepant from professional ethics, and specifically, the APA Code (2002). But, the issue is far from clear. It is a situation where experts must try to reconcile any conflict or tension between professional ethics and what may be legally permitted (Shuman & Greenberg, 2003).[2] Our position is the APA Code does not preclude reviewers from expressing a wide range of opinions on the data contained in the evaluator's case file and evidence that may be heard in court based on the three parts of Rule 9.01, so long as there is sufficient and adequate basis for doing so (e.g., Rule 9.01(a)). These opinions need to be closely attached to the data reviewed concerning behavioral patterns and function and not be loosely applied to a person's general characteristics or a diagnosis. A colleague remarked to us that this rule (9.01(c)) seemed to be ambiguous if a reviewer could opine about individuals' characteristics (but not patterns of behaviors or events or results of psychological testing). We believe 9.01, as interpreted in its plain language, is not ambiguous if the three parts are interpreted in concert, as APA clearly intended since part (b) refers to part (c).

The APA Code, Rule 9.01(a) states:

> Psychologists base the opinions contained in their recommendations, reports, and diagnostic or evaluative statements, including forensic testimony, on information and techniques, sufficient to substantiate their findings (p. 1071).

We suggest this is the primary guidance for all expert opinions by psychologists. They need to be informed opinions based on adequate data.

The APA Code, Rule 9.01(b) states:

> Except as noted in 9.01(c), psychologists provide opinions of the psychological characteristics of individuals only after they have conducted an examination of the individuals adequate to support their statements or conclusions (p. 1071).

We suggest the field of psychology has focused almost exclusively on this part of 9.01 as if the third part of the rule did not exist. Part (b) has been the "Holy Grail" of psychological evaluation, and we do not disagree with the position that personal evaluation is extremely important. The question here and for the field is whether it is a *necessary* condition to form opinions about individuals, behavior patterns, and issues to be considered to have directly assessed the person. Personal or direct evaluation is what psychologists generally do, but there are many contexts where opinions are called for without a personal, direct examination. For example, could the psychologist, after reviewing a school psychology report with all the testing and observational data available, not render an opinion if the student had a learning disability? The third part of 9.01 (and as noted in part "b") shows that it was the intent of APA that direct examination should not be a necessary condition to opine about an individual. This is not an ambiguous statement.

The APA Code, Rule 9.01(c) states:

> When psychologists conduct a record review or provide consultation or supervision and an individual examination is not warranted or necessary for the opinion, psychologists explain this and the sources of information on which they based their conclusions and recommendations (p. 1071).

To demonstrate that the main issue in any discussion about what opinions a forensic mental health expert can and should express (or a clinical psychologist/psychotherapist for that matter) is the adequacy of the foundation for the opinions and whether or not the opinion is free of bias or other distorting influences. The forensic context of the retrospective assessment of mental states in litigation (Simon & Shuman, 2002) is based the review of documents and records, or perhaps collateral interviews as well. Ogloff and Otto (1993) point out "Effective mental health assessments typically require the participation of the examinee ... However, some legal questions arise that necessitate an examination of a decedent's mental state prior to his or death" (p. 607). Forensic experts have long been asked to and permitted to opine about the mental states of the deceased in testamentary capacity evaluations. When the question before the court concerns the state of mind of an individual when he executed a will and whether "undue influence" or "coercive persuasion" was placed on that person by another person (Simon, 2002a), then the court naturally would like some assistance from psychology or psychiatry. The person is obviously not directly evaluated. The expert reviews records and statements of third parties about the circumstances facing the person when the will was executed and the behaviors of the person accused of manipulating the vulnerable elderly person, now deceased. In order for the expert to render an opinion on the decedent's state of mind, he or she has to believe there was the necessary and sufficient information available. Another similar forensic example involves the assessment of a deceased state of mind to determine the cause of death on the issue of whether it was a suicide, perhaps at the request of an insurance company. The evaluation involves a "postmortem suicidal risk assessment" and opinions about the cause of death and the person's state of mind, including or related to the person's psychological characteristics and clinical diagnosis, if any (Simon, 2002b). In other contexts, psychologists are called upon to perform a "psychological autopsy" and express an opinion sometimes for the purpose of criminal prosecution (Ebert, 1987; Ogloff & Otto, 1993).

We suggest there is an ethical foundation for reviewers, especially if they are combining instructional testimony with a work product review, to offer opinions, not just about methodology and about the synchrony between the evaluator's opinions and data. We assert the quality and appropriateness of an expert's opinions concerns the sufficiency of the database for the expressed opinion. We believe the APA Code clearly permits reviewers to issue considered and well-reasoned opinions about mediate issues and specific interpretations of the meaning of data. Generally, the reviewer will not want to offer opinions that are explicitly about a person's psychological characteristics or to suggest a diagnosis. However, for example, if the evaluator suggested a parent had a narcissistic personality disorder and this was a reason for limiting parenting time, then the reviewer might opine if the data supported the evaluator's opinion on the clinical diagnosis. Conversely, if the evaluator gave little weight to a pattern of behavioral data and psychological testing that clearly was consistent with a narcissistic personality disorder, including data on its impact on parenting behaviors, then the reviewer would want to address that issue. To refrain from saying there were overwhelming data in support of a hypothesis that the parent's behaviors and testing were consistent with a personality dysfunction and that there were indications of impaired parenting function would seem to be ignoring the elephant in the room and not being helpful to the court. Out of deference to ethical etiquette, however, the retaining attorney would want to phrase the question to the expert in hypothetical form. When reviewers come to know a family through an intensive review of a child custody case file, we suggest, the reviewer comes to understand the family and the important issues. We suggest reviewers recognize that generally there really is no benefit to offering opinions on specific characteristics of the parents or children, or to explicitly offer a diagnosis, but there can be benefit to offering opinions in response to hypothetical questions on a variety of mediate, or focused issues that will be helpful to the court.

We suggest there is not a logical or discernible difference between the evaluator responding to hypothetical questions, and the reviewer doing the same based on the same, sufficiently detailed dataset and fact pattern. The evaluator has the benefit of direct observation that yields nonverbal information, but if there is an exact record in the case file (e.g., electronic recordings), then this difference largely disappears. When an evaluator goes to court to testify it may have been many months or over a year since the evaluation was completed. Our experience is that the evaluator-expert witness not infrequently is vague or rusty about details in the data. The difference between the thorough reviewer and evaluator can start to diminish. The reviewer may know the evaluator's data better than the evaluator. We do acknowledge the important difference between an evaluator and reviewer, but they should be operating from the same dataset. We do not recommend that reviewers should opine specifically about parties' psychological diagnoses or characteristics, but hypothetical questions are very legitimate as established by the highest court. We feel reviewers can help clarify for the court the interpretation of the evaluator's data and the issues in the case. A useful perspective is that the evaluator almost always *reviews* documents and records as part of the custody evaluation, and the reviewer always *evaluates* the child custody report and case file.

Courts do not want the hands of helpful experts to be tied so they feel constrained to not address the data and issues. In most cases, where there have been problems with the forensic quality of the custody evaluation identified, the reviewer should provide (1) a balanced analysis of the strengths and weaknesses of the evaluation; (2) reinforce the opinions of a quality evaluation or identify any fatal flaws; (3) be able to opine about mediate issues on the correct interpretation of data on salient issues; (4) respond to hypothetical questions about a fact pattern that resembles the case-specific data that the reviewer has learned; (5) provide instructional testimony and case analysis; (6) offer opinions about a person's psychological characteristics or diagnosis only in a hypothetical form; (7) not opine on the ultimate issues about custody, even if presented in hypothetical form; and, (8) be able to provide opinions about interpreting the data reviewed on behavioral patterns, meaning of events and actions, psychological testing, and records. We suggest the psychologist-forensic reviewer needs to be able to directly interpret and opine on data that are reviewed if there is an adequate and sufficient basis for those opinions. The advisability on what opinions are offered by the reviewer expert probably should come from a pragmatic analysis of the context of the case and the extent of information available to the reviewer-expert just as *Daubert* (1993) proposes a pragmatic analysis for trial court judges. The ethical reviewer should recognize when there is a sufficient knowledge base for the opinions expressed.

PRACTICE TIPS

1. Custody evaluators need to mindful of the standard of practice, professional guidelines and standards, and the professional literature in approaching every case.
2. Custody evaluators should anticipate the possibility that they will be subject to a work product review as they design and conduct every evaluation.

3. Reviewers need to conduct their practice with keen mindfulness about being an ethical reviewer while acknowledging the reality that they will be perceived as biased and aligned with the position of the retaining attorney.
4. Reviewers should strive to be perceived by the court as aligned with the data in the case, or giving high quality and insightful analysis.
5. Helpfulness to the court should be the guiding principle for reviewers. Helpfulness depends on conducting an objective review of the custody report and giving balanced, candid feedback to the retaining attorney.
6. Reviewers need to discuss with the retaining attorney the expectations concerning the consulting service to be provided as a testifying expert. Will the reviewer help prepare questions for his or her direct examination? Discuss trial strategy? Educate the attorney, and subsequently the court, about relevant research on issues in the case? Help prepare questions for the evaluator or other witnesses in order to facilitate the elicitation of the "best testimony" for the court?
7. Reviewers need to be mindful that the attorney-client and work product privileges will disappear when they are identified as a testifying expert. This fact means the reviewer needs to be mindful on what types of written work product is produced as part of consulting with the attorney.
8. Reviewers and evaluators need to vigilantly follow the ethical standards that require their opinions to be based on sufficient and the necessary information in order to answer the questions for the court.

SUMMARY

The forensic roles that experts fulfill and the services they provide in child custody litigation were described. These roles are custody evaluator, reviewer of the evaluator's work product, provider of instructional-educational testimony, and the non-testifying forensic consultant. We recommended that emphasis be placed on the types of forensic services that experts provide instead of roles since experts provide multiple services in most cases. We distinguished between testifying and non-testifying experts. Emphasis was placed on the role of the reviewer of the work product of the child custody evaluator. It is essential that reviewers first conduct an objective review of the custody report before providing any consultation services. Helpfulness to the court and objectivity in analysis was presented as the guiding principle for both the neutral court evaluator and the retained expert in the role of reviewer. Instructional testimony is sometimes the focus of a retained, testifying expert, but is found to some degree in all expert testimony. How the retained expert in the role of reviewer can establish credibility depends on the adherence to the principles of helpfulness and objectivity. Judges will recognize balanced and well-reasoned analysis and testimony and the accuracy of opinions in light of the data and evidence in the case. Other dimensions of expert testimony and issues concerning the ethics of providing testimony in the role of reviewer were discussed: (1) what opinions reviewers can express; (2) if reviewers can consider data not gathered by the evaluator, including courtroom testimony; (3) the need to help the court assess the reliability and validity of an evaluator's methodology and approach in light of legal standards and rules of evidence; (4) application of the APA Code of Ethics to reviewer services and testimony; and, (5) the function of reviewers to assist in monitoring custody evaluations as forensic quality control as opposed to seeing reviewers as hired guns. The article reminds the reader of the need for ethical review work in child custody cases based on professional standards, and also, the oath that each testifying expert swears to before taking the witness chair.

NOTES

1. While standard of practice requires custody evaluators to create and maintain a very high quality case record, this often is not the case. Interview notes often are approximations or narrative and not verbatim. The only "true interview data" would be collected by electronic recording, which is easy to accomplish, but few evaluators do so.

2. Professional organizations have weighed in is support of the position of requiring direct, personal examination of a person to offer opinions about psychological-psychiatric diagnosis in the form of guidelines, standards, and amicus briefs in appellate cases, American Psychological Association, American Psychiatric Association, and American Bar Association.

REFERENCES

Ackerman, M. J. (2001). *Clinician's guide to child custody evaluation*, 2nd ed. New York: John Wiley.

American Psychological Association (APA). (1994). Guidelines for child custody evaluations in divorce proceedings. *American Psychologist, 49,* 677–680. doi:10.1037/0003-066X.49.7.677

American Psychological Association (APA). (2002). Ethical principles of psychologists and code of conduct. *American Psychologist, 57,* 1060–1073. doi:10.1037/0003-066X.57.12.1060

American Psychological Association (APA). (2009, February). Guidelines for child custody evaluations in family law proceedings. Unpublished manuscript, Approved by APA Council of Representatives.

Association of Family, and Conciliation Courts (AFCC). (2006, May). *Model standards of practice for child custody evaluation.* Madison, WI: Author; Martindale, D. M., Martin, L., Austin, W. G. et al. (2007). Model standards of practice for child custody evaluation. *Family Court Review, 45*(1), 70–91.

Atkinson, J. (2010). The law of relocation of children. *Behavioral Sciences & the Law, 28,* 563–579. doi:10.1002/bsl.944.

Austin, W. G. (2009). Responding to the call to child custody evaluators to justify the reason for their professional existence: Some thoughts on Kelly and Ramsey

(2009). *Family Court Review*, *47*(3), 544–551. doi:10.1111/j.1744-1617.2009. 01272.x

Austin, W. G., & Drozd, L. M. (2006, June 1). Custody evaluation and parenting plans for relocation: risk assessment for high conflict or partner violence. Workshop presented at Association of Family and Conciliation Courts, 43rd Annual Conference, Tampa, FL.

Austin, W. G., Flens, J. R., & Kirkpatrick, H. D. (2010, June 3). *Gatekeeping and child custody evaluation: Theory, measurement & applications*. Association of Family and Conciliation Courts, 47th Annual Conference, Denver, CO.

Austin, W. G., Kirkpatrick, H. D., & Flens, J. R. (in press). The emerging forensic role of work product review and case analysis in child access and parenting plan disputes. *Family Court Review*, *49*.

Austin, W. G., Kirkpatrick, H. D., & Flens, J. R. (submitted). The psychology of reviewing the work product of a colleague for the court in child custody evaluation.

Bala, N. (2004). Assessments for postseparation parenting disputes in Canada. *Family Court Review*, *42*(3), 485–510. doi:10.1111/j.174-1617.2004.tb00665.x

Bala, N. (2005). Tippins and Wittmann asked the wrong question: Evaluators may not be "experts," but they can express best interests opinions. *Family Court Review*, *43*, 554–562. doi:10.1111/j.1744-1617.2005.00054.x

Barefoot v. Estelle, 463 U.S. 880, 103 S.Ct. 3383 (1983).

Bow, J. N., & Quinnell, F. A. (2004). Critique of child custody evaluations by the legal profession. *Family Court Review*, *42*(1), 115–127. doi:10.1111/j.174-1617. 2004.tb00637.x

Committee on Ethical Guidelines for Forensic Psychologists (1991). Specialty guidelines for forensic psychologists. *Law and Human Behavior*, *15*(6), 655–665. doi:10.1007/BF01065858

Daubert v. Merrell Dow Pharmaceuticals, Inc. 509 U.S. 579 (1993).

Ebert, B. W. (1987). Guide to conducting a psychological autopsy. *Professional Psychology: Research and Practice*, *18*(1), 52–56. doi:10.1037/0735-7028.18.1.52

Elrod, L. D., & Dale, M. D. (2008). Paradigm shifts and pendulum swings in child custody: The interests of children in the balance. *Family Law Quarterly*, *42*(3), 381–418.

Emery, R. E., Otto, R. K., & O'Donohue, W. T. (2005). A critical assessment of child custody evaluations. *Psychological Science in the Public Interest*, *6*(1), 1–29. doi:10.1111/j.1529-1006.2005.00020.x

Federal Rules of Evidence (FRE). (2008). Thomson/West.

Galatzer-Levy, R. M., Kraus, L., & Galatzer-Levy, J. (Eds.). (2009). *The scientific basis of child custody decisions*, 2nd ed. New York: Wiley.

Gould, J. W. (2006). *Conducting scientifically crafted child custody evaluations*, 2nd ed. New York: Guilford.

Gould, J. W., Kirkpatrick, H. D., Austin, W. G., & Martindale, D. (2004). A framework and protocol for providing a forensic work product review: Application to child custody evaluations. *Journal of Child Custody: Research, Issues, and Practices*, *1*(3), 37–64. doi:10.1300/J190v01n03_04

Gould, J. W., & Martindale, D. A. (2005). A second call for clinical humility and judicial vigilance. *Family Court Review*, *43*, 253–259. doi:10.1111/j.1744-1617. 2005.00025.x

Gould, J. W., & Martindale, D. A. (2007). *The art and science of child custody evaluations*. New York: Guilford.

Hage, J. (1972). *Techniques and problems of theory construction in sociology*. New York: John Wiley.

Heilbrun, K. (2001). *Principles of forensic mental health assessment*. New York: Kluwer Academic/Plenum Publishers.

Hickman v. Taylor, 329 U.S. 495 (1947).

Holloway v. State, S.W.2d 479 (Tex. App. 1981).

In re Marrriage of Seagondollar, 139 Cal.App. 4th 1116, 43 Cal.Rptr 3d. 575 (2006).

Kelly, J. B. (1997). The best interests of the child: A concept in search of meaning. *Family and Conciliation Courts Review*, *35*, 377–387. doi:10.1111/j.174-1617.1997.tb00480.x

Kelly, J. B., & Emery, R. (2003). Children's adjustment following divorce: Risk and resilience perspectives. *Family Relations*, *52*, 352–362. doi:10.1111/j.1741-3729.2003.00352.x

Kelly, J. B., & Johnson, M. P. (2008). Differentiation among types of intimate partner violence: Research update and implications for interventions. *Family Court Review*, *46*(2), 476–499. doi:10.1111/j.1744-1617.2008.00215.x

Kelly, R. F., & Ramsey, S. H. (2009). Child custody guidelines: The need for systems-level outcome assessments. *Family Court Review*, *47*(2), 286–303. doi:10.1111/j.1744-1617.2009.01255.x

Kirkpatrick, H. D. (2004). A floor, not a ceiling: Beyond guidelines – An argument for minimum standards of practice in conducting child custody and visitation evaluations. *Journal of Child Custody*, *1*, 61–76. doi:10.1300/J190v01n01_05

Martin, L. (2005). Commentary on "empirical and ethical problems with custody recommendations—to recommend or not recommend. *Family Court Review*, *43*(2), 242–245.

Martindale, D. A. (2005). Confirmatory bias and confirmatory distortion. *Journal of Child Custody: Research, Issues, and Practices*, *2*, 33–50. doi:10.1300/J190v02n01_03

Martindale, D. A. (2006a). Consultants and role delineation. *The Matrimonial Strategist*, *24*, 3–5.

Martindale, D. A. (2006b). The Oz illusion: The expert behind the curtain. *The Matrimonial Strategist*, *24*, 5–6.

Martindale, D. A. (2010). Psychological experts and trial tactics: The impact of unarticulated contingencies. *The Matrimonial Strategist*, *28*(8), 5–6.

Martindale, D. A., & Gould, J. W. (2007). Countertransference and zebras: Forensic obfuscation. *Journal of Child Custody*, *4*(3/4), 69–76. doi:10.1300/J190v04n03_05

Martindale, D. A., & Gould, J. W. (2008). Evaluating the evaluators in custodial placement disputes. In H. Hall (Ed.) *Forensic psychology and neuropsychology for criminal and civil cases* (pp. 527–546; 923–935). Boca Raton, FL: Taylor & Francis.

Melton, G. B., Petrila, J., Poythress, N. G., & Slobogin, C. (2007). *Psychological evaluations for the courts, 3rd ed.* New York: Guilford.

Mnookin, J. L., & Gross, S. R. (2003). Expert information and expert testimony: A preliminary taxonomy. *Seton Hall Law Review*, *34*, 139–185.

Mnookin, R. H. (1975). Child custody determination: Judicial functions in the face of indeterminacy. *Law and Contemporary Problems, 39*(3), 226–293. doi:10.2307/1191273

Newmark, L., Harrell, A., & Salem, P. (1995). Domestic violence and empowerment in custody and visitation cases. *Family and Conciliation Courts Review, 33*, 30–62. doi:10.1111/j.174-1617.1995.tb00347.x

Ogloff, J. R. P., & Otto, R. K. (1993). Psychological autopsy: Clinical and legal perspectives. *Saint Louis University Law Journal, 37*(3), 607–646.

People v. Wilson, 133 A.D.2d 179 (N.Y. App. 1987).

Pickar, D. (2007). Counter transference bias in the child custody evaluator. *Journal of Child Custody, 4*(3/4), 45–68. doi:10.1300J190v04n03_06

Rohrbaugh, J. B. (2008). *A comprehensive guide to child custody evaluations.* New York: Springer.

Rollerson v. United States, 343 F.2d 269, 274 (D.C. Cir. 1964).

Shuman, D. W., & Greenberg, S. A. (2003). The expert witness, the adversary system, and the voice of reason: Reconciling impartiality and advocacy. *Professional Psychology: Research and Practice, 34*(3), 219–224. doi:10.1037/0735-7028.34.3.219

Shuman, D. W., & Sales, B. D. (1998). The admissibility of expert testimony based on clinical judgment and scientific research. *Psychology, Public Policy, and Law, 4*(4), 1226–1252. doi:10.1037/1076-8971.4.4.1226

Simon, R. I. (2002a). Retrospective assessment of mental states in criminal and civil litigation: A clinical review. In R. I. Simon & D. W. Shuman (Eds.), *Retrospective assessment of mental states in litigation* (pp. 1–20). Washington, DC: American Psychiatric Association.

Simon, R. I. (2002b). Murder, suicide, accident, or natural death? In R. I. Simon & D. W. Shuman (Eds.), *Retrospective assessment of mental states in litigation* (pp. 135–154). Washington, DC: American Psychiatric Association.

Simon, R. I., & Shuman, D. W. (Eds.). (2002). *Retrospective assessment of mental states in litigation.* Washington, DC: American Psychiatric Association.

Stahl, P. (1996). Second opinions: An ethical and professional process for reviewing child custody evaluations. *Family and Conciliation Courts Review, 34*, 386–395. doi:10.1111/j.174-1617.1996.tb00428.x

Stahl, P. M. (2005). The benefits and risks of child custody evaluators making recommendations to the court. *Family Court Review, 43*(2), 260–265. doi:10.1111/j.1744-1617.2005.00026.x

State of North Carolina v. Daniels, 446 S.E.2d 298 (N.C. 1994).

Tippins, T., & Wittmann, J. (2005). Empirical and ethical problems with custody recommendations. *Family Court Review, 43*, 193–222. doi:10.1111/j.1744-1617.2005.00019.x

Tippins, T. M. (2009). Expert witnesses and consultants. *The Matrimonial Strategist, 27*(3), 1, 3–4.

Ver Steegh, N. (2005). Differentiating types of domestic violence: Implications for child custody. *Louisiana Law Review, 65*, 1379–1431.

Consulting with Attorneys: An Alternative Hybrid Model

S. MARGARET LEE

Independent Practice, Mill Valley, California

LORIE S. NACHLIS

Independent Practice, San Francisco, California

This article discusses the recent expansion of the roles assumed by mental health professionals within the field of family law. In the past, mental health professionals working within the family law system, most frequently, worked as neutral child custody evaluators. More recently, articles and conference presentations have described the emergence of other roles such as "review expert," "consulting trial expert," "witness support," or collaborative divorce "coach." In these newer roles, the mental health professional is retained, not as a neutral, but as an expert for one parent. This article will address the ethical implications present in this work. In addition, the authors will further expand the field by describing the various functions of a "hybrid consulting expert," the unique contribution provided by this collaboration, and the ethical and practical dilemmas that it creates.

Mental health professionals are providing an increasing array of services to courts, attorneys, and families, including serving as experts, consultants, mediators, and coaches. Traditionally, the Mental Health Professional was often cast in the role of a neutral, appointed by the court to evaluate a particular family and make recommendations regarding the custody of the children. The Mental Health Professional as custody evaluator has been the subject of many books and articles (Gould, 1998; Stahl, 1999). Numerous guidelines have been developed to define the procedures of the Mental

Health Professional (MHP) as custody evaluator and to address the potential ethical issues that may arise (AFCC, 2006; APA, 1994, 2009; California Rules of Court, 1999/2003/2004/2007/2010).

With the increase in the number of forensic psychologists, psychiatrists, social workers, and therapists involved in child custody matters, we are seeing an expansion of the roles fulfilled by these professionals. Some of the roles include:

1. Acting as a "review expert" for one side or the other: In this role, the MHP is usually retained by the attorney to review and critique the evaluation performed by another MHP and, possibly, provide an opinion regarding the evaluator's work to the court at a trial (Martindale, 2006; Gould, Kirkpatrick, Austin, & Martindale, 2004);
2. Providing litigation assistance and consultation to one side or the other at various stages of the proceedings of the custody dispute: This "behind the scenes" consultation typically involves educating the attorney regarding the psychological aspects of the case, assisting the attorney in the development of trial strategy, and drafting questions for use in the examination of expert witnesses; and
3. Acting as a coach to a parent (Hobbs-Minor & Sullivan, 2008; Coates, Flens, Hobbs-Minor, & Nachlis, 2004; Burrows & Buzzinotti, 1997): In this role, the MHP provides support to a parent during a child custody evaluation. This role is also referred to as "witness support."

As the possible roles for MHPs expand within the field of family law, there is a need to examine how to maintain the ethical and professional responsibilities of a MHP while working within a system that has a different set of rules, responsibilities, and ethics. The complexity of the roles and the absence of guidelines have been of concern to those operating in this field. The Association of Families and Conciliation Courts has recently convened a task force to explore the ethical and professional problems that may be present by the assumption of various roles within the legal field.

An Alternative Model: Hybrid Consulting

Most of the roles previously mentioned are assumed by MHPs during the litigation phase of a case. With the hybrid consulting model, the MHP may perform a variety of roles, sometimes blurring the lines between them. The involvement of the MHP typically begins early in the case, sometimes immediately after or concurrently with the retention of the attorney. One of the primary goals of this collaboration is the thorough exploration of potential alternatives to resolution by traditional adversarial means, including an examination of the risks and benefits of each alternative. The hybrid consultant will perform the dual, and seemingly inconsistent, functions of assisting with settlement while simultaneously assisting in the development of litigation strategy in the event that litigation is necessary. In addition, the hybrid consultant provides a psychological perspective and education to the attorney and the parent throughout her involvement in the case.

The attorney, MHP and the parent jointly commit to pursue a course of action that is mindful of the best interests of the children involved. The team proceeds based upon the understanding that in most situations, the children's interests will be served if their parents are able to cooperatively share the tasks of parenting. This acknowledgement, that is, that litigation frequently polarizes families and potentially injures, sometimes irreparably, the parents ability to co-parent, provides the motivation to seek alternatives to litigation while simultaneously recognizing that at times resolution by judicial decision cannot be avoided.

This model presents ethical challenges for the MHP, specifically in terms of maintaining objectivity, avoiding inappropriate dual roles, and doing no harm (APA, 2002/2010). In this article, the ethical considerations are based on the American Psychological Association's Ethics Code (APA, 2002/2010, 2009); however, the issues, if not the exact codes, are seen as applicable to all mental health professionals working in family law cases.

An Understanding of the Judicial System

Our legal system is an adversarial system. "The adversary system is based on the assumption that the truth of a controversy will best be arrived at by granting the competing parties, with the help of an advocate, an opportunity to fight as hard as possible" (Johnston and Lufrano, 2002).

> The unleashing of litigation in its full fury has done cruel, grave harm and little lasting good. It has helped sunder some of the most sensitive and profound relationships of human life: between the parents who have nurtured a child; between the healing professions and those whose life and well-being are entrusted to their care...It seizes on former love and intimacy as raw materials to be transmuted into hatred and estrangement. It exploits the bereavement that some day awaits the survivors of us all and turns it to an unending source of poisonous recrimination. It torments the provably innocent and rewards the palpably irresponsible. It devours hard-won savings and worsens every animosity of a diverse society. (Olson, 1991).

Law schools emphasize litigation as the primary method of dispute resolution such that lawyers are trained to think first about litigation when consulted by a client. Students are required to take multiple classes that are geared to mastering the system of litigation ("Changing law schools," 1997). Although most schools now offer multiple courses in mediation and negotiation, very few courses are offered that specifically relate to family law. In addition, many of the traditional methods of ADR are often highly structured and contentious. Many of the courses in family law that are offered to future attorneys address issues of child custody from a litigation point of view, emphasizing the rights of the parents over the best interests of the child. As with contracts, torts, estates, civil procedure, and other courses that are offered in law school, students learn about child custody by studying the cases that have reached the highest courts through rounds of litigation.

In this society based upon laws, parents who are unable to resolve disputes concerning parenting issues, resort to a system of laws in which each parent's interest is frequently represented by an attorney who may know the system, but rarely understands the needs of the child. The attorney's education and training focuses on litigation as the go-to system available to resolve the client's problem. Law school curriculums do not usually train attorneys to assess the psychological issues underlying most custody disputes or to consider the psychological issues when weighing the risks and benefits of potential methods of resolution. Attorneys are not trained to assess a child's best interest or the detrimental impact that parental conflict has on children's post-divorce development.

Most attorneys are taught to be zealous advocates for their clients. The use of attorneys in today's world to resolve disputes is not much different than the use of jousters in the middle ages.

Mahatma Ghandi, a trained attorney, stated in his autobiography:

> I saw that the litigation, if it were persisted in, would ruin the plaintiff and the defendant, who were relatives and both belonged to the same city...[I]t might go on indefinitely and to no advantage of either party...In the meantime, mutual ill-will was steadily increasing. I became disgusted with the profession. (Katsh, 1986).

For many years, a discussion has ensued within the family law legal community about the effectiveness as well as the destructiveness of the use of traditional litigation methods in which each side is represented by attorneys charged with zealously advocating the interests of his or her clients. This discussion has been motivated by an acknowledgement that the break up of a marriage involves complicated emotional problems that impact not only the couple, but also the children, those working with the children, friends, and extended family members. In addition, the expenses associated with the breakup of the marriage can be astronomical and beyond the reach of many.

In 2000, the American Academy of Matrimonial Lawyers amended their Bounds of Advocacy, acknowledging that the concept of zealous advocacy may be harmful and stated that an effective advocate means "considering with the client what is in the client's best interests and determining the most effective means to achieve that result. The client's best interests include the well being of children, family peace, and economic stability" (AAML, 2000). This broader view of the client's interests removes what some have experienced as an ethical dilemma and has introduced into the role of the attorney the need to educate the client about the impact of decisions on the needs of his or her child, not only when considering the resolution of custody issues, but also when considering the impact on the children of the fight regarding financial issues.

The lawyer must competently represent the interests of the client, but not at the expense of the children. The parents' fiduciary obligations for the well being of a child provide a basis for the attorney's consideration of the child's best interests consistent with traditional advocacy and client loyalty principles (AAML, 2000).

Limitations of the Adversarial System

The legal system moves very slowly and inefficiently. It is common in many jurisdictions for evaluations to take months, for hearings to be repeatedly postponed or for custody trials to involve non-sequential, partial days of testimony with frequent delays and rescheduling, resulting in trials stretching over months. When dealing with young children, the "custody fight" can come to impact a quarter or half of their lifetime. For older children, many are aware that their life is in limbo: Will they be living here or there, going to this school or that one, will their time with one parent continue to be supervised or in some cases will there be any contact at all with one parent? The lack of clarity can result in children being anxious about how their lives will eventually be structured.

In a system which traditionally declares a winner and a loser, cases dealing with the custody of a child are sometimes litigated in such a way that the prize is the child. Which parent gets the child may have financial ramifications that sometimes motivate an aggressive fight. When the child is the prize, one side may find it beneficial to manipulate the system by delaying the proceedings. As the disputing process extends, parents can become increasingly polarized and adversarial, increasing the likelihood that the children will be brought into the middle of the conflict. A child's adjustment to divorce is highly correlated to the degree to which they are exposed to their parents' conflict, particularly if the conflict is about them (Amato, 2001; Kelly, 2000; Kelly & Emery, 2003).

It is not our intention in this article to propose that the legal system be eliminated as a source for resolution of disputes. We recognize that there are situations in which a neutral trier of fact must, for the benefit of the child, sort through competing evidence and make a determination. Cases requiring a finding of fact, such as serious allegations of domestic violence and child abuse, often are best served by having the court involved. Cases such as severe child alienation may also require that the court remain involved over time to monitor parents' compliance with court orders or to provide backing for a Parent Coordinator (Special Master) (Sullivan & Kelly, 2001).

When considering alternatives to the legal system, it should be acknowledged that there is no alternative that can be chosen which removes the power of the court to resolve an issue should the alternatives chosen fail to resolve the matter. The court remains as an option and can be a powerful tool to encourage settlement outside of court. By seeking processes that are alternative to the court process, the professionals are frequently searching for solutions that may go beyond what could be provided by the courts and that are tailored to a specific family's needs and lifestyle.

Definition and Examples of Hybrid Consulting with a Team Approach

Some alternatives to litigation are well established and involve clearly delineated functions and processes. These alternatives include child custody mediation and collaborative law. The hybrid consulting model includes the flexibility to adopt various functions and processes, depending on the specific case, that may change as the case proceeds. Prior to exploring the goals and possible functions incorporated in this model, a few examples may help to illustrate the scope and diversity of how an attorney, parent, and MHP can work as a team.

Case Examples

CASE EXAMPLE 1. MOVING A FAMILY FROM ONGOING CONFLICT AND DISPUTE TOWARDS A SOLUTION

Susan, a 40 year old mother of two children, consulted with an attorney five years following her marital separation. She was very concerned about her 10-year-old daughter, Molly, a child with attentional and learning difficulties. During the past years, the parents had disputed the appropriateness of the schedule they had agreed upon, offered different interpretations of their agreement, and every holiday and vacation involved tense negotiations. Molly was reported to be having difficulties going between homes and managing her parents' different parenting styles. The school reported that Molly was not happy at school and was beginning to show signs of lowered self-esteem. Susan was concerned that the lack of a consistent structure was impacting both Molly's academic progress and her sense of self. Susan's attorney immediately retained a MHP as a consultant. The MHP reviewed school records, previous evaluations and both parents' declarations, and met together with the attorney and her client. Based on the material reviewed, it appeared clear to the MHP that regardless of which parent's perspective was more accurate, this family would benefit from a child custody evaluation that would help clarify what would be an appropriate parenting schedule for this special needs child. The attorneys were able to negotiate an agreement to have Molly begin seeing a therapist and were able to agree on a specific therapist (not without some wrangling and dispute). However, the father strongly opposed an evaluation, expressing his belief that it was unnecessary. The attorney and the MHP decided to invite the father and his attorney to a meeting where the MHP explained her reasoning as to why an evaluation would be helpful. This effort was, in fact, unsuccessful. The attorney filed a motion asking the court to order an evaluation. The MHP provided a declaration in support of the requested relief. In her declaration, she outlined the material she reviewed, described in general terms the needs of children with attentional difficulties and learning disabilities, and set forth the reasons why an evaluation was warranted in this family. The court ordered an evaluation.

CASE EXAMPLE 2. MANAGING THE HARM CAUSED BY A POORLY PERFORMED
CHILD CUSTODY EVALUATION, SEEKING ALTERNATIVES TO LITIGATION AND
ASSISTING WITH THE LITIGATION

Mother and Father were never married. Prior to the birth of Hannah, they negotiated an arrangement whereby Father would visit with Hannah at Mother's residence. After a few months, Father wanted to visit with child away from Mother. Mother was uneasy, but agreed. By the time Hannah was two, Father was demanding frequent overnights. Mother agreed to overnights, but a dispute concerning the frequency and duration of the overnights could not be resolved and a custody evaluation was ordered by the court. The evaluator raised concerns about the Father's ability to be attuned to the child's needs, as well as about his credibility, but ultimately recommended a schedule of increasing overnights.

During the next year, Father continued his demand for ever increasing time with the child, requiring frequent court appearances, was very critical of Mother, and declared over and over again how perfectly well the child was doing when in his care. Mother reported that the child was deteriorating in her care. She was not sleeping well, clinging to mother, and crying hysterically on the days that she was to go to Father's home. A limited scope evaluation was ordered. This evaluator saw the child present very well in Father's care and become emotionally deteriorated when with Mother, both prior to and after the visits with Father.

Father had successfully painted the picture of Mother being the cause of any distress experienced by the child. The court announced its intention to order an equal timeshare of Hannah when Hannah was four years old.

Mother consulted with a new attorney who immediately retained a mental health professional to meet with mother, review the previous evaluations, declarations, and the communications between the parents. The MHP wrote a declaration in support of Mother's position and offered hypotheses that should be explored that were alternatives to Mother being the cause of the child's distress. None of these alternatives had been explored by the evaluators. The MHP suggested that a failure to explore these alternatives and proceed with an equal timeshare could potentially expose the child to a significant risk of harm.

The court ordered a new evaluation. During this evaluation, the Father was abusive to the evaluator and to the child's therapist. Individuals who had witnessed Father frightening the child and demeaning the mother to the child responded to requests by the evaluator for information. The evaluator found Mother's descriptions of the child's behaviors to be credible and that Mother was floundering based upon an inability to protect her child.

Father rejected the recommendations of the neutral evaluator and a 6-day trial eventually was held. The MHP worked with Mother and the Attorney to prepare for trial. She assisted with the preparation of the examination of Father's expert. At the conclusion of the trial, Father's visitation with Hannah was ordered to be supervised.

CASE EXAMPLE 3. ASSISTING A FATHER AND HIS ATTORNEY TO
UNDERSTAND THE CHILDREN'S DEVELOPMENTAL NEEDS AND SET REALISTIC
TIMESHARE EXPECTATIONS

George hired an attorney shortly after his wife left him. She accused him of having had an affair. Wife took the two children, aged 2 and 4 years, and prevented any contact between the father and his children for three weeks. George was demanding a 50/50 parenting plan despite the fact that he was the sole wage earner in the family and worked a 60-hour work week. He was also insisting that his wife become gainfully employed immediately. The attorney brought in a MHP as part of the team, both to help her understand her client and to explore the attachment and developmental issues involved in the case.

The attorney's initial concern entailed whether George would be able to focus on his children's best interests given her observation of his anger. The attorney arranged a meeting involving the attorney, George and the MHP. During this three-hour meeting, the MHP interviewed George about the marital history, the separation and the children, as well as his thinking about his proposed parenting plan. Following the meeting, the MHP opined to the attorney that although George was clearly very angry, this was likely a situational reaction to the separation. This opinion was based on his ability to demonstrate a clear understanding of his children and the fact that his angry feelings significantly escalated when talking about the betrayal by his wife.

The attorney and the MHP decided to approach George in an educational manner. The MHP explained that his emotional reaction to the separation was quite normative but was interfering with his thinking clearly about his children's needs. The MHP recommended that George enter into psychotherapy (with another MHP). This was followed with education about attachment issues in very young children and about the structuring of a parenting plan that would support the children's attachment relationships with their mother while providing him with the opportunity to become a more involved father.

The team developed a proposal for shared legal custody and a parenting plan that would gradually increase father's time with his children and allow his wife to stay home until the youngest child entered preschool. The proposal was rejected, based upon mother's reported belief that George lacked parenting skills and the proposal involved too much time away from her. Fortunately, mother's attorney had also hired a MHP well versed in young child development. Following a day of discussion and negotiation where the two MHPs talked with each other, the respective parents and the attorneys (all present), an agreement was reached that both MHPs believed would support the children's relationships with both of the parents. The attorneys were then able to formalize the agreement. In this case, it was clear that it was through the efforts of both attorneys and both MHPs, which this case not only settled but that the settlement supported the children's developmental needs. This meeting also was a first step in helping these two parents learn to work in a more cooperative, co-parenting manner.

These case examples illustrate some ways a MHP can provide assistance to the attorney and parents by helping them explore approaches to resolution, by recommending services and interventions, and by educating them in a variety of areas. One of the advantages of the team approach is the flexibility to find a workable solution for a specific family that involves the mental health professional's assumption of various roles during the course of her involvement. This approach is most successful when the attorneys for both parents value mental health input and are interested in finding alternative routes to settlement aside from a courtroom resolution. The cohesive element involved in this team approach is a commitment made by all team members to the children's best interests.

Goals of Alternative Hybrid Consulting

The following are some goals that frequently can be achieved more effectively through the use of alternative and hybrid consulting models:

1. Helping a family achieve stable post-separation functioning: For many, the period immediately post-separation is fraught with anger and fear. Parents are called upon to make decisions at a time when many of them are incapable of making good decisions. It is at this time that many seek the assistance of attorneys and are too often guided to the court where solutions are fashioned that rarely meet the specific needs of the family.

For some families, that path to the courthouse becomes one that is well traveled, creating a group of family court litigants sometimes referred to as "frequent fliers." Whether a family goes down a path of trying to find a workable solution to divorce that serves their children's needs and their own needs or whether they go down a war path, can be influenced by their attorney's or the MHP's actions. Case Example 3 illustrates a situation where the father's unrealistic thinking was addressed and the process helped the parents begin to work together. The negotiations and education involved in the process also modeled for the parents a successful approach to resolving future problems.

2. Moving beyond a win-lose perspective: Alternatives to court can help parents move beyond the concept of having a winner and a loser. Particularly in those jurisdictions where custody and support are interdependent, the stakes are higher. Since the amount of support is tied to the amount of time spent with the children, some parents may be motivated to win more or less time in order to impact financial obligations and benefits.

   Even when financial outcomes are not a motivating factor, a "win-lose" attitude entrenches parents in their position, focusing them on building a better case rather than looking for flexible, thoughtful and individualized solutions. Discussions involving the attorney and the MHP emphasize the children and their needs, not how a parent can gain an advantage.

3. Helping a parent and his or her litigation team to maintain the focus on the child during the course of the litigation: The idea of litigation returns us to the concept of winning and losing. Strategic decisions are being made regularly. The litigation team maps out a strategy and revises that strategy with a conscious effort made to adopt the winning approach. During that time, it is very easy to focus on winning, or beating the other side, rather than on what is necessary to meet the needs of the child. Litigation is about parties and sides. It is important to keep in mind even during the course of litigation that it is about the child and the child's best interests. This consulting model helps the attorney and the parent understand the interests of the child when developing a strategy for litigation. Case Example 1 involved developing a strategy to accomplish the goals of getting the child in therapy and finding an avenue wherein the child's special needs could be addressed, that is, having a child custody evaluation ordered. Case Example 2 also addressed educating the parent and the attorney as well as assisting with the litigation.

4. Educating the parent and the team: The parent is the only member of the team who knows the child. In assisting the team to focus on the child's best interest, the mental health consultant provides education concerning developmental issues, the impact of divorce on children's development, as well as more specifically, the impact of the parent's and the team's actions on the child's best interests. A consulting MHP also brings a different training and attitude to the legal process. The MHPs are trained to use

their clinical skills to hold and weigh conflicting information, without having to immediately direct a course of action. The MHPs are trained to observe nuances, to strive to maintain objectivity even in the face of strong emotions, and are alert to the long-term impact of one's actions. The MHPs training provides a balance to that of the attorney. All three cases involve some degree of deliberation, thinking through alternative courses of action, and attempting various solutions short of court action. Despite these efforts, involvement of the court was required in two cases (1 and 2).

The Hybrid Consulting Model and the Establishment of the Team

In what we refer to as the team or collaborative approach, the MHP is typically brought into the matter by the attorney at, or very near, the time that the attorney is first retained. The attorney may, in fact, want psychological input about the prospective client in order to assist the attorney in making the decision to accept or reject the case. The attorney may also want to have a better understanding of her client's psychological dynamics from the onset of the case in order to work more effectively with the parent while maintaining objectivity and appropriate boundaries. The MHPs contract is with the attorney and the parent is made aware that the attorney, not the parent, is the MHP's client. The attorney determines whether meetings will be three-way meetings or whether the consultant will meet directly with the parent without the attorney present. There must be informed consent in terms of the parent knowing that what is told to the consultant is not confidential, i.e., it will be shared with the attorney.

The MHP is a member of a team consisting of the parent, attorney and the MHP. When participating as a member of the team, the MHP is lending a psychological perspective and education throughout the process while melding that perspective and education with (1) the attorney's knowledge of the law, the court system, and opposing counsel; and, (2) the parent's knowledge of the child as well as of the other parent.

As a member of the team, the MHP performs various functions, depending on the specific case. The MHP participates in analyzing all of the available facts and formulating the issues that may need to be addressed in order to successfully resolve the case. This is not unlike the function that is frequently performed by a litigation consultant where the consultant may be asked to address case strategy after reviewing motions and declarations. During such a review, when issues such as possible domestic violence, substance abuse, child abuse and severe child alienation arise, the MHP is able to assess whether the concerns may be valid or fabricated or confused and provide that feedback. When there is a possibility of such serious events having occurred, the MHP can help identify how best to further evaluate the degree of risk and/or what interventions would reduce the risk. In addition to actively participating in the analysis of the facts, the MHP typically provides the attorney and the parent with education about the psychological elements of the case and how they can best be assessed or managed.

Most MHPs who participate in this type of consultation are experienced Child Custody Evaluators. They bring to the process, skills for developing multiple hypotheses and an understanding of how to collect data that will confirm or disconfirm the various hypotheses. Once the facts of the case have been laid out and analyzed, the MHP can provide feedback in terms of the pros and cons of various parenting plans that might be appropriate, what possible interventions could address the identified problems, and whether or not there needs to be a full evaluation so that all the needed data can be collected in a neutral manner.

The next step in the process often involves discussing the strategy by which these goals can be reached. For example, if the information collected suggests that the children are upset and are being placed in the middle of their parents' dispute, a reasonable plan would be to get psychotherapy for the children and to have the parents involved in co-parent counseling as the legal case is proceeding. This may be accomplished through a discussion between the parents or their attorneys. However, if there is resistance, the attorney may file a motion with an accompanying declaration written by the MHP, articulating the data supporting the need for the interventions (see Case 1). If both "sides" have consulting MHPs, the attorneys may decide that having the MHPs talk with each other could lead to resolution on some issues (see Case 3).

Continued Consultation when a Child Custody Evaluation has been Agreed to or Ordered

After an initial approach to the case has been determined, the MHP consultant will likely continue involvement with the attorney and the client. If a Child Custody Evaluation has been ordered, the attorney and the consultant are likely to discuss choosing between possible evaluators, their areas of expertise or any known biases, in addition to the potential evaluator's general competence. How long a given evaluator typically takes to complete an evaluation may be a critical factor in some cases. The MHP may also consult directly with the parent. She may help the parent better understand the litigation process; the evaluation process; and she may suggest strategies to the parent that will help the child deal with issues that arise from living within a shared parenting environment during the course of an evaluation. This latter function may be very similar to what has been described as "coaching" or "witness preparation" in the literature.

At the completion of the evaluation, the consultant and the attorney will review the evaluation, discuss what approach to take with the evaluation, that is, accept the findings and recommendations, try to fine-tune the recommendations, or oppose the evaluation. The process of reviewing the evaluation and determining whether it is an adequate evaluation is similar to what is done by a "review expert." A review expert is a MHP who is retained to review another professional's custody evaluation, critique said evaluation, possibly provide his/her own analysis of the data collected, and provide the attorney and parent an opinion regarding the quality/usefulness of the evaluation.

If the evaluator's recommendations are opposed, the attorney frequently will hire a second consultant to act as a testifying expert. The original consultant will likely continue to assist the attorney as a trial consultant, to help develop deposition and trial questions for the experts.

If the evaluation is seen as an adequate but contrary to the wishes of the client, the MHP will help the team consider options, including accepting the recommendations. This may involve, in a limited way, helping the parent process their difficult emotions to enable them to take in what the evaluator has said and to help the parent respond to criticisms in a proactive, constructive manner. If the parent is destabilized by the results, the consultant will likely encourage the parent to enter therapy to explore and process their feelings, as the consultant cannot slip into being a treating therapist for the parent.

Following some evaluations, an opportunity for settlement may exist. Settlement efforts may be informal or involve a judicial settlement meeting with the judge. Settlement efforts may include the MHP. There are situations when MHPs hired by either side of the dispute will work together to facilitate settlement and help make adjustments to the recommendations and there are situations when the MHP participates in judicial settlement conferences, usually with the permission of both attorneys and/or the judge.

When the MHP is involved in settlement efforts, either with the other attorney or those involving the judge, they can help the participants maintain a focus on the child, help maintain a problem-solving attitude, and reduce polarization. When two MHPs are involved, it is helpful to engage in thoughtful and respectful discussions and avoid the pull to become polarized and adversarial, or to become competitive. Observing the professionals interact in such a way can be a model for how resolution can occur and how conflict can be managed without becoming destructive. Some judges have commented on the advantages of having multiple perspectives but this can only occur when the MHPs maintain a neutral stance, respectful with each other.

Continued Consultation without Evaluation

In cases that do not proceed to a Child Custody Evaluation, the attorney and the MHP discuss how to negotiate with the other attorney to find an acceptable resolution. If a resolution cannot be reached through negotiations via the attorneys, the MHP will help determine whether or not the court system will be utilized, taking into consideration the potentially negative impact that litigation will have on the family. Factors such as who is the opposing counsel will likely influence the chosen process.

Advantages of the Hybrid Consulting Model

This hybrid model, where a MHP is partnered with the attorney and the parent, allows for tremendous flexibility. It also incorporates and utilizes two distinctly different areas of expertise in order to find creative solutions for families. The work towards resolution is always within the "shadow of the law" (Mnookin & Kornhauser, 1979); thus, when developing strategies and actions, consideration is given to how the court might view the evidence and ultimately rule. However, working outside of the court allows for flexibility and tailored solutions.

By participating as an equal member of the team, the Mental Health Professional is receiving information that is not being screened by either the attorney or the parent. The advantage that this provides is that the MHP is less likely to end up in a position where she is advocating a position that is based upon facts previously selected by the attorney or the parent who has hired her. As a result, the credibility of the MHP is enhanced, decreasing the risk that the court would dismiss the opinions offered by the MHP as a result of bias. Another factor that helps the MHP maintain a scientific and objective, and, therefore, ethical stance is the constant focus on the child's best interest combined with a vigilant awareness that one only has partial information. It is essential for the MHP to avoid being pulled into "group think." By maintaining this focus and awareness, the MHP can help the attorney maintain an objective perspective of their client.

The hybrid consulting model involves collaboration between the parent, attorney and the MHP. It is different from the role that the MHP assumes in a case that proceeds pursuant to the rules and requirements of Collaborative Law. When a case is a Collaborative Law case, the parties, attorneys, and experts commit to transparency and agree that if a resolution cannot be achieved through the collaborative law process, none of the professionals involved can participate in the court process. In the hybrid process, decisions are made and strategy is discussed with the understanding and the possibility that a resolution may be imposed upon this family by a judge. Another difference between the hybrid consultant and the collaborative law coach is the issue of who is the client. In the hybrid model the attorney is the client, whereas in collaborative law, the parent is the client. The team approach results in the parent being educated about both the psychological as well as the legal ramifications of his or her decisions and actions.

A variety of considerations can impact the attorney's decision to bring in a MHP to work in a consulting or hybrid role. The financial resources available to the client are probably the most limiting factor. The available financial resources may make the use of consultants impossible, may limit the role solely to a few hours of consultation, or limit the role to solely that of a testifying expert. When a MHP is brought into a case, regardless of the role, the MHP's contract is with the attorney. The work of the MHP is protected by the attorney work product privilege from discovery by the other side in the event the matter goes to court, so long as the MHP does not become a testifying witness. The more involved the MHP is with the client and the attorney, the more important this shield becomes.

Professional and Ethical Issues

Using a MHP in a hybrid role raises risks for the attorney if ultimately the case ends up in court. The MHP with the most knowledge is someone who generally cannot be used in court. This is particularly so if the MHP has been part of the team. Litigation is not a transparent process; it is a strategic process in which the goal is to prevail. The MHP who has been part of the team has also been part of the development of strategy. If that person testifies, all of the information provided to the MHP is now available to the other side. If a court proceeding takes place, a MHP who has not had access to the information and probably to the parent is going to be required. This adds to the cost of an already costly process. It is essential to carefully define at all stages of the engagement the role that it is expected that the MHP will fulfill. Will the MHP be a consulting expert or a testifying expert; and if a testifying expert, should that person have any contact with the parent based upon the possibility that the MHP's opinion can be tainted by only having contact with one side?

Although a MHP in this model may perform various functions and use skill sets developed as a forensic practitioner, a developmental psychologist, and a clinician, this model need not involve multiple roles that impact objectivity and effectiveness. The APA Ethics Code, section 3.05a (2002/2010) in part states that "... A psychologist refrains from entering into multiple relationships if the multiple relationship could reasonably be expected to impair the psychologist's objectivity, competence, or effectiveness in performing his or her functions as a psychologist, or otherwise risks exploitation or harm to the person with whom the professional relationship exists." It is extremely important that the role and the possible functions within that role be clearly articulated and agreed upon through informed consent prior to commencing this work. In cases where one has had multiple relationships, the MHP is usually precluded from testifying not only because of the access that he or she has had to the development of legal strategy, but also because there is a greater likelihood that objectivity cannot be assured and that there would at least be an appearance of bias.

In addition, the opinion of the MHP who has only met one parent, or perhaps neither parent, and certainly not the children, is necessarily limited by this lack of data. She can opine about a course of action and or interventions that should be pursued. Her opinion is limited by the possibility that the party for whom she is working has not been truthful. In any public statements, whether in court or in settlement efforts, it is critical that the MHP clearly defines the basis for any opinion and the limits of that opinion (APA Ethics Code, section 9.01). There is an inherent dilemma in this work as the "best interests of the children," as seen by the MHP, is intrinsically limited by not having evaluated the child directly. In any discussion of what the MHP sees as the best interests of the child, there needs to be a clear articulation of the limits of that understanding. As noted in Section VI. H of the Division 41 of the APA "Specialty Guidelines for Forensic Psychologists" (APA, 1992), "Forensic psychologists avoid giving written or oral evidence about the psychological characteristics of particular individuals when they have not had an opportunity to conduct an examination of the individual adequate to the scope of the statements, opinions or conclusions to be issued. Forensic psychologists make every reasonable effort to conduct such evaluations. When it is not possible or feasible to do so, they make clear the impact of such limitations on the reliability and validity of their professional products, evidence or testimony."

The MHP, although working within a legal arena, remains bound by her own ethics code. She remains a mandated reporter. The parent working with the MHP as part of the team, may disclose to the MHP that he or she has witnessed behaviors between the other parent and the child which necessitates a referral to Child Protective Services, despite the client's and the attorney's desire to keep CPS out of the process. Or, the parent may describe abusive behavior that he or she has directed at the child, requiring a child abuse report.

When working with a parent who is being evaluated, the line between helping a parent become a better parent and coaching a parent to look better for the evaluator is sometimes not that obvious. Although permissible to support the client going through an evaluation and permissible to help a parent respond appropriately to their child's behavior, helping them "fake good" is not permissible. Also, when explaining the evaluation process to the parent, it is permissible to describe the process of psychological testing and what the tests measure but it is not permissible to help the parent "practice" the tests or take any other actions that would compromise test security (APA Ethics Code, Section 9.11, 2002/2010).

If the MHP maintains a commitment to take no action that is or may be contrary to the best interests of the child (as understood by the available data), the MHP will assist the attorney in making choices that are based upon a realistic view of the client and the client's relationship with the child as well as with the other parent. The MHP must avoid the pull towards polarization or a biased view of either parent.

Given the fact that this role involves multiple functions and potentially multiple roles, it is imperative that the MHP not only be vigilant in her effort to avoid biases, but she must also not become an advocate in a manner that impairs objectivity or removes the focus from the best interests of the child. The MHP's training to carefully weigh data, to look for both confirmatory and dis-confirmatory data and to think through complex, multi-factored situations, is critical to maintaining a non-adversarial stance and to avoiding premature actions. Maintaining a constant awareness that being involved in multiple tasks can impact one's objectivity is a challenge that must be met. One important way to avoid being pulled into nonobjective, polarized thinking is to see oneself as essentially "representing the child." This focus on the child is also helpful when disagreements arise between the parent and the attorney or when engaging with the attorney/client and opposing counsel. This work involves a lot of self-monitoring on the part of the MHP and is only successful when the attorney and the MHP have a respectful relationship. As is true for many complex tasks performed by MHPs, obtaining consultation from well trained colleagues can be useful in maintaining objectivity and clarity.

The complexity of this role and the range of skills required mean that the MHPs performing this work should be quite experienced in a number of areas. This role requires knowledge of child development, family dynamics, and forensic principles. A hybrid consultant needs to have significant familiarity with the court system and its legal underpinnings. Finally, a hybrid consultant needs to understand ethical issues, not just the codes, but how some actions can be damaging to individuals, to one's credibility, or to one's profession.

Further Steps in Developing this Role

As new roles for MHPs emerge in the area of family law, understanding their usefulness, advantages, and pitfalls occurs through professional discussion and increasingly refined thinking. Consultants involved in reviewing/critiquing evaluations, trial consultants, witness support, collaborative law coaches, and hybrid consultation have different goals and functions resulting in various limitations and ethical challenges. Meaningful debate regarding the ethical issues and dilemmas that might arise from the combination of the functions and actions within the hybrid consulting model should occur. A continuing dialogue between attorneys and MHPs must continue so that the each discipline understands the perspectives, motivations, and the principles to which the other must adhere.

REFERENCES

Amato, P. (2001). Children of divorce in the 1990's: An update of the Amato and Keith (1991). A meta-analysis. *Journal of Family Psychology, 1*, 355–370. doi:10.1037/0893-3200.15.3.355

American Academy of Matrimonial Lawyers (AAML). (2000). *Bounds of advocacy.* Chicago, IL: American Academy of Matrimonial Lawyers.

American Psychological Association (APA). (1994). Guidelines for child custody evaluations in divorce proceedings. *American Psychologist, 47,* 1597–1611.

American Psychological Association (APA). (2002, 2010). *Ethical principles of psychologists and code of conduct.* Adopted in 2002 and amended in 2010. Washington, DC: American Psychological Association.

American Psychological Association (APA). (2009). *Guidelines for child custody evaluations in family law proceedings.* Washington, DC: American Psychological Association.

American Psychological Association, Division 41 (APA). (1992). *Specialty guidelines for forensic psychologists.* Washington, DC: American Psychological Association.

Association of Family and Conciliation Courts (AFCC). (2006). *Model Standards of Practice for Child Custody Evaluation.* Madison, WI: Association of Family and Conciliation Courts.

Burrows, R., & Buzzinotti, E. (1997). Legal therapists and lawyers: Care-giving partnerships for the next century. *Family Advocate, 19*(4), 33–36.

California Rules of Court, Rule 5.220. Amended effective January 1, 2010; adopted as rule 1257.3 effective January 1, 1999; previously amended and renumbered effective January 1, 2003; previously amended effective July 1, 1999, July 1, 2003, January 1, 2004 and January 1, 2007.

Coates, C., Flens, J., Hobbs-Minor, E., & Nachlis, L. (2004, October). Coaching clients for custody evaluations: Is it ethical? *Workshop presentation for Association of Family and Conciliation Courts, Sixth International Symposium on Child Custody Evaluations,* Nashville, Tennessee.

Changing law schools to make less nasty lawyers. (1997, Winter). *Georgetown Journal of Legal Ethics, 367.*

Gould, J. (1998). *Conducting scientifically crafted child custody evaluations.* Thousand Oaks: Sage Press.

Gould, J., Kirkpatrick, H. D., Austin, W., & Martindale, D. (2004). Critiquing a colleague's forensic advisory report: A suggested protocol for application to child custody evaluations. *Journal of Child Custody, 3,* 37–64. doi:10.1300/J190v01n03_04

Hobbs-Minor, E., & Sullivan, M. (2008). Mental health consultation in child custody cases. In L. Fieldstone & C. Coates (Eds.) *Innovations in interventions with high conflict families* (pp. 159–186). Madison: Association of Family and Conciliation Courts.

Johnston, R., & Lufrano, S. (2002). The adversary system as a means of seeking truth and justice. *35 J. MARSHALL L. REV.* 147, 147 (2002).

Katsh, M. (1986). *Taking sides: Clashing views on legal issues 14,* (2d. ed. 1986) (quoting Mahatma Gandhi's autobiography). Guilford, CT: Dushkin Pub. Group/Brown & Benchmark Publishers.

Kelly, J. B. (2000). Children's adjustment in conflicted marriage and divorce: A decade review of the research. *Journal of Child and Adolescent Psychiatry, 39*(8), 963–973. doi:10.1097/00004583-200008000-00007

Kelly, J. B., & Emery, R. (2003). Children's adjustment following divorce: Risks and resilience perspectives. *Family Relations, 52*(4), 352–362. doi:10.1111/j.1741-3729.2003.00352.x

Martindale, D. A. (2006). Consultants and further role delineation. *The Matrimonial Strategist*, *24*, 4, 4ff.

Mnookin, R. H., & Kornhauser, L. (1979). Bargaining in the shadow of the law: The case of divorce. *88 Yale Law Journal* 950. doi:10.2307/795824

Olson, Walter K. (1991). The litigation explosion: What happened when American unleashed the lawsuit 2.

Stahl, P. (1999). *Complex Issues in custody evaluations*. Thousand Oaks, CA: Sage.

Sullivan, M., & Kelly, J. B. (2001). Legal and psychological management of cases with an alienated child. *Family Courts Review*, *39*(3), 299–315. doi:10.1111/j.174-1617.2001.tb00612.x

Psychological and Legal Considerations in Reviewing the Work Product of a Colleague in Child Custody Evaluations

H. D. KIRKPATRICK

Independent Practice, Charlotte, North Carolina

WILLIAM G. AUSTIN

Independent Practice, Lakewood, Colorado

JAMES R. FLENS

Independent Practice, Brandon, Florida

This article has three primary objectives: 1) to examine what the authors believe are some important psycholegal and ethical considerations for work product reviews of a child custody evaluation; 2) to make suggestions to custody evaluators and retained reviewers to incorporate the concept of "helpfulness to the court" as a fundamental, guiding principle; and 3) to offer some suggestions about how and why a custody evaluator might derive some positive value from a competent and ethical review of his or her work product. The role of a reviewer of the work product of the court's appointed child custody evaluator is becoming more common in custody litigation. The functions and ethics of this evolving role are discussed. The inherent tension between a retained reviewer's obligation to provide ethical and helpful testimony to the court, while in the role of a retained expert, is examined. The psychological perspectives of both evaluator and reviewer are presented. This article discusses the commonly held, but erroneous, belief that a psychologist (as a retained reviewer) has an ethical duty to discuss his/her concerns with the psychologist whose work was reviewed. The legal and ethical reasons why the APA ethics code (2002) does not apply to review work are presented.

ROLE OF THE REVIEWER IN CHILD CUSTODY CASES

With increasing frequency, forensic mental health professionals are involved in child custody disputes and litigation to provide consultation and expert testimony after the completion of a child custody evaluation. An evolving role is that of a retained reviewer to provide an analysis and opinion of the quality of the child custody evaluation process, including a review of the evaluator's written report and the evaluator's methodology. The custody evaluator's role is to provide a neutral, objective, and impartial evaluation of the parents and children, to address the pertinent referral questions, and to make recommendations to the court based on the psychological best interests of the child. The evaluator is either court-appointed or appointed by a consent order. As a consultant/educator to the court, the child custody evaluator's goal is to address the referral questions in a manner most helpful to the court, while adhering to all applicable forensic, legal, and ethical guidelines.

The reviewer's role is distinctly different from the child custody evaluator's role. The obvious difference is the reviewer is retained by one party to critique/review the work of the court-appointed custody evaluator. Nevertheless, as will be discussed, even though the reviewer is a retained expert whose fees are paid by one party's attorney and whose testimony (if given) is expected to be helpful to that attorney and his or her client, being *helpful* to the court also should be the overriding goal of a reviewer. We are advocating this goal should be foremost on a reviewer's mind, just as it should be on the custody evaluator's mind. Although retained by one party, a reviewer is a specific type of expert consultant to the court, ideally providing information, and reasoning to the court that aids the court's deliberations about the child's best interests. We argue that, once a review has been completed and the reviewer has identified some significant problems with the underlying child custody evaluation, the reviewer has an obligation not only to be helpful to the retaining party but also to the court. As discussed in the following, on rare occasions, a reviewer might be retained by one party to give testimony about the strengths and weaknesses of a custody evaluation. A competently done cross-examination of a retained reviewer should be able to elicit opinions about a custody evaluation's strengths. A reviewer who only presents the "bad" and the "ugly" findings to the retaining attorney and presents the same slanted testimony to the court, accurately, will be viewed as a "hired gun." We argue a reviewer, as a retained expert, should give balanced testimony, based on an ethical and defensible review of a custody evaluation. Once a retained reviewer is declared as an expert witness for one party, we believe the reviewer has an obligation to be helpful to the court (Austin, Dale, Kirkpatrick, & Flens, 2011). The principle of helpfulness, as we use it here, means the work product and/or testimony of a forensic expert should a) be true to the data and issues in the case and b) present an honest, balanced, objective analysis for the court.

While the experience of reviewers may be that it is not uncommon to encounter poor quality in child custody evaluations, there is an absence of research on general quality. Survey studies have been conducted on the procedures used by evaluators (Ackerman & Ackerman, 1997; Bow & Quinnell, 2001) and how evaluators approach special issues such as domestic violence (Bow & Quinnell, 2003). One of Bow's surveys examined the quality of custody reports (Bow & Quinnell, 2002) and another surveyed the concerns of lawyers and judges about custody evaluations and evaluators (Bow & Quinnell, 2004). Another study, using a small sample of convenience, studied the forensic quality of the reports and evaluations (Horvath, Logan, & Walker, 2002). Kelly and Ramsey (2008) recently called for research on the effectiveness of custody evaluations or a cost/benefit analysis of what evaluations really provide in light of their use of court and financial resources. Austin (2009), in commenting on Kelly and Ramsey, suggested that steps to provide forensic quality control, such as work product reviews, would be a means to increase the benefit to the courts and litigating parents. Kelly and Ramsey's ambitious research proposal would include an assessment of the quality of custody evaluations (Kelly & Ramsey, 2008). The available research indicates there are reasons to be concerned about the general quality of custody evaluations, not surprisingly, given the wide variance in the training and experience of evaluators to conduct what may be the most complex and difficult of all forensic mental health evaluations. There also are no established criteria or dimensions for assessing the quality of custody evaluations. We suggest quality can be assessed in terms of a) methodology, b) knowledge of law and research, c) data collection, d) data interpretation, e) the correspondence between the evaluator's opinions and the underlying data, and f) the evaluator's awareness and use (when appropriate) of the standards, guidelines, and parameters of practice. One of the authors of this article has argued there are certain minimum standards one should consider in conducting a child custody evaluation (Kirkpatrick, 2004). We also believe balanced reviews can provide rich data about the quality of custody evaluations.

To gain a better perspective on the role of a reviewer in the child custody context, it is helpful to be aware of the common use of retained experts, consultants, and rebuttal experts in civil litigation. The "tension in the roles experts are expected to play is fundamental to the way in which experts are used in the legal system" (Shuman & Greenberg, 2003). The tension results from a duality in their role, i.e., who retains them for what purpose and their ethical duty to appear helpful and objective. For understandable reasons, it would appear the retained expert "starts out in a hole" on the issue of perceived credibility. She must overcome this uphill climb so the court will come to see the expert's testimony as accurate, unbiased, and helpful and thus be persuaded by the retained expert's testimony on the issues in dispute. We believe it is optimal for a retained expert to give testimony that is viewed by the court as being true to the data and issues of the case, i.e., perceived as being aligned congruently with the data and providing ethical expert testimony, rather than perceived as singularly aligned with the retaining attorney's advocacy position (Tippins, 2009; Shuman & Greenberg, 2003).

To state the obvious, a retained expert does not have the same standing as the court's appointed expert. We see three reasons for this difference in status: 1) the retained expert is hired by one side, and, until declared as a testifying expert witness, her role is cloaked in the attorney-client work privilege; 2) the retained expert's role and task do not give her access to some of the original data, e.g., the retained expert never interviews the parties, child(ren), or collaterals; 3) the retained/reviewing expert's task is entirely different from the task of the custody evaluator. A retained review of a custody evaluator's work is not a "second opinion." To stay with the metaphor of the uphill climb the retained expert faces, the retained expert will only achieve credibility with the court by adhering to all applicable standards, guidelines and practice parameters, by articulating to the court the limits of the reviewer's task and findings, and by focusing on the strengths and weaknesses of the custody evaluator's methodology and written report.

Ethical guidelines in forensic psychology require the retained expert to provide objective analysis and balanced testimony, meaning properly addressing alternative views of the data and alternative hypotheses, no matter who is paying the expert's fees. The Specialty Guidelines (1991) are usually cited to support this position. We believe presenting balanced and objective testimony is the only tenable position for a reviewer to take if she wants the court to take her seriously:

> In providing forensic psychological services, forensic psychologists take special care to avoid undue influence upon their methods, procedures, and products, such as might emanate from the party to a legal proceeding by financial compensation or other gains. As an expert conducting an evaluation, treatment, consultation, or scholarly/empirical investigation, the forensic psychologist maintains professional integrity by examining the issue at hand from all reasonable perspectives, actively seeking information that will differentially test plausible rival hypotheses (Committee on Ethical Guidelines for Forensic Psychologists, 1991, p. 341).

The structure and outline of how to conduct a competent work product review have been previously described (Gould, Kirkpatrick, Austin, &

Martindale, 2004; Stahl, 1996; Martindale & Gould, 2008), but more research needs to be done. At this point, there are no standards of practice or consensus on how to define the role of reviewer.[1] Issues involved in the role of reviewer vs. consultant have recently been discussed (Austin, Dale, Kirkpatrick, & Flens, 2011; Tippins, 2009; Martindale, 2010). The role of reviewer can be thought of as an "emerging forensic role" (Austin et al., in press). Yet, at the same time, courts are becoming more aware that consultants and reviewers are being used with increasing frequency. Second evaluations in custody cases, or a second court-appointed expert, are rare in some jurisdictions (i.e., California), but commonplace in others (i.e., Colorado). Although, as stated above, a work product review is not a "second opinion," but a review can be obtained in lieu of a second evaluation and can be helpful to the court.

Little has been written about the role of a reviewer in the professional guidelines or standards pertaining to child custody evaluations. The APA child custody guidelines (American Psychological Association, 1994) identified the role of a reviewer as appropriate: "[o]r a psychologist may be asked to critique the assumptions and methodology of the assessment of another mental health professional" (III. 8.). The Model Standards for Child Custody Evaluation (AFCC, 2007) has one small section or rule, on the role of reviewer (Rule 8.5). It addresses the issue of dual roles so the reviewer should not have a prior relationship with or meet with the litigants or members of the litigants' families. This is a general statement and does not address the issues of how the reviewer's role is defined or the functions inherent in the role, e.g., reviewing work product, consulting, providing general testimony on research and professional issues.

The Code of Conduct by the American Psychological Association (2002) anticipates that psychologists will sometimes be called upon to review documents and records and issue opinions (Rule 9.01(c)), which is the essential task of the reviewer role when the reviewer becomes a testifying expert based on a review of child custody report and case file. Rule 9.01(c) states:

> When psychologists conduct a record review or provide consultation or supervision and an individual examination is not warranted or necessary for the opinion, psychologists explain this and the sources of information on which they based their conclusions and recommendations (p. 1071).

This rule presumably was not designed in 2002 to address the role of reviewer in child custody cases, but it is a generic rule for the many psycho-legal contexts in which psychologists practice where they are asked to review records and issue opinions about the data and issues that were reviewed and interpreted. The rule is not meant to replace evaluations and the opinions based on directly gathering data on the person or persons in question.

For example, an insurance company may retain a clinician to review hospital records to determine if there was sufficient basis for the diagnosis being used for billing for services. This rule follows and is an exception to the rule (9.01(b)) that opinions should not be expressed about persons who have not been personally evaluated and about whom there is not an adequate basis for the opinions expressed:

> Except as noted in 9.01(b), psychologists provide opinions of the psychological characteristics of individuals only after they have conducted an examination of the individuals adequate to support their statements or conclusions (p. 1071).

Both of the above rules are part of, or follow from the initial rule or standard (Rule 9.01(a)), there should be the necessary and sufficient data before expressing opinions or recommendations:

> Psychologists base the opinions contained in their recommendations, reports, and diagnostic or evaluative statements, including forensic testimony, on information and techniques, sufficient to substantiate their findings (p. 1071).

When a retained forensic expert reviews the work product of the court's appointed child custody evaluator, the purpose is to conduct an objective assessment of the forensic quality without any preconception that the purpose is to find only weaknesses or deficiencies in the evaluation. Our profession requires that the review should be a fair, balanced, and accurate assessment of the overall quality—meaning, identifying the strengths as well as weaknesses. An objective assessment is the *sine qua non* of review work, as noted by the few published articles on the structure and issues in a competently conducted work product review (Gould et al., 2004; Austin et al., in press) and forensic ethical guidelines (Specialty Guidelines, 1991). Shuman and Greenberg (2003) point out that the same issue and pressure on the retained expert exists in other types of forensic mental health cases. These authorities warn that retained experts "may perceive they must choose between integrity and advocacy," but this is a "false choice" (p. 219), because it is possible to define the retained expert role in a way "that permits experts to be concurrently ethical, persuasive, impartial, and helpful" (p. 219) to the court and the retaining attorney. Shuman and Greenberg (2003) also point out that retained experts may be permitted by courts to give testimony in such a way that compromises their professional ethics, so the testifying expert has the responsibility of alerting the court to any conflict between law and ethics. They go on to propose an "alternative, integrated approach" to providing ethical testimony in the role of a retained expert based on (1) attending to the need to be competent or well trained; (2) providing relevant testimony; (3) developing a perspective on maintaining neutrality in the midst of adversarial advocacy; (4) guarding against bias and providing a balanced analysis including the consideration of alternative hypotheses; and (5) being candid and forthright about the basis for one's opinions and the limitations of the data and method. Shuman and Greenberg (2003) remind us that the system of civil litigation depends on and routinely uses multiple retained experts to educate and inform courts. This view of experts applies to the role of a reviewer in custody cases.

The following sequence of steps outlines the process and stages of the ethical work product review of a child custody evaluation:

1. The expert is contacted by the retaining attorney, who requests the expert review a child custody report and provide candid feedback on the quality of the evaluation and report. Typically, the expert is asked specifically to address whether the recommendations and ultimate issue opinions are supported by the data in the report. The prospective reviewer anticipates the legitimate advocacy position of the retaining attorney.

2. If the expert agrees to accept the task, the expert sends the retaining attorney a "retainer contract" (or "letter of understanding") spelling out the nature of the services to be provided, the expert's understanding of what she is being retained to do, and emphasizing the work product review will be an objective, but limited, assessment. The contract or letter of understanding stresses that any future consultation or testimony services will be discussed only after the objective review is completed. It is prudent to obtain an appropriate non-refundable retainer in full prior to providing any review work. The contract or letter of understanding articulates the expert's recognition of the two distinct phases of expert consultation: 1) the role and tasks of a non-testifying reviewer, whose consultation and findings are confidential and protected by the attorney work-product privilege; and 2) the role and tasks of an expert witness, whose consultation and findings (including any written material) are not protected, are not confidential, and are discoverable, under the rules of evidence.

3. The expert conducts an ethical and objective review, analysis, and assessment of the child custody report without succumbing to any expectations or agenda that only weaknesses of the report will be addressed. A balanced analysis of the strengths and weaknesses is conducted on the procedures, data collection, data analysis, and formulation of opinions as articulated in the written report. The reviewer examines whether the opinions formulated seem to correspond with the underlying data based just upon a critical reading and analysis of the custody report.

4. There appears to be consensus that experts should not engage in consultation on a case and then shift to the role of trying to conduct an objective work product review (Heilbrun, 2001). The expert would then

already be aligned with the advocacy position and probably would not be viewed as credible by the court. This is the central reason we emphasize that the retained expert tell the retaining counsel—upfront and in writing—that the review will be conducted in an ethical and objective manner.

5. The reviewer provides candid, cogent feedback to the attorney on the strengths and weaknesses of the written report. If an analysis of the report suggests there are serious deficiencies and what appear to be fatal flaws, which far outweigh the evaluation's strengths, e.g., the evaluation may not be helpful to the court or might be misleading or biased, then this opinion is communicated to the retaining counsel at this time, after which the attorney and reviewing expert discuss her future involvement in the case.

6. Decisions are made about the expert's future role and forensic function, or services to be provided. The pros and cons of the reviewer's opinions being used in testimony are discussed. If the reviewer opines that the custody evaluation report was of significantly poor quality and possibly inaccurate in its opinions and recommendations, then the attorney likely will want the reviewer to become a testifying expert and to provide some degree of trial consultation services. This decision point puts the reviewer at the threshold of stage two of the expert reviewer role.

7. Next, if the attorney wants the expert to conduct a comprehensive work product review, the attorney (through discovery) will arrange to obtain the evaluator's case file so the reviewer can conduct a thorough review of the file and relate it to the custody report.

8. The attorney and expert will define the consultation part of the role and services to be provided. This may include assistance in preparing questions for the custody evaluator's cross-examination and the reviewer's direct examination. The attorney may view this consultation as helpful to his advocacy for the client's position. The ethical expert will have the perspective that assistance in addressing issues in the case and eliciting testimony will facilitate better quality of evidence being made available to the court. Therefore, the retained expert concurrently is being helpful to the court and to the retaining counsel.

9. The attorney and expert will decide if a written report, based on the review, is necessary and helpful. The attorney will be focused on legal strategy and it will be his or her call to ask the expert to prepare a rebuttal report to buttress the expected testimony, or decide not to prepare a report. In some jurisdictions, a report would be required.

10. The attorney and expert will discuss if the testimony will only consist of a review of the quality of the evaluation and report, or if instructional testimony on the research and professional literature relevant to issues in the case will be combined with the review testimony. This would be a hybrid role of a work product review and professionally relevant

education on the issues, or more accurately a combination of forensic services. All expert testimony has an educational component for the court to some degree (Mnookin & Gross, 2003). Many child custody evaluators discuss the literature and research on salient issues as part of their testimony and in their reports. Reviewers should be prepared to discuss the relevant literature and research, if requested to do so by the retaining attorney, and if appropriate, while offering testimony to the court. A reviewer should foresee she will be asked to discuss relevant literature and research under cross-examination.

PSYCHOLOGICAL PERSPECTIVES OF THE REVIEWER

As the reviewer heads toward becoming a testifying expert (and identified as such), there should be psychological sensitivity on her part to anticipate how the child custody evaluator likely will respond to being reviewed. The evaluator will probably view the process as a "critique," highlighting potential flaws in the evaluation because the reviewer probably would not be testifying if he or she did not feel there were serious deficiencies questioning the accuracy of the evaluator's opinions and recommendations. The reviewer should also anticipate some evaluators will view the review as an "attack." Occasionally, though, the reviewer may be asked to supplement or reinforce the evaluator's opinions and, basically, give testimony that the evaluation was sound and the data supported the evaluator's interpretations and opinions.

The ethical and competent reviewer will approach her task with the mindset that expressed opinions critical of a colleague's work product will be constructive criticism of the evaluation, not of the evaluator, with the overall objective of being helpful to the court. The ethical reviewer who takes a balanced approach to his or her role will want the testimony and/or report to be persuasive, unbiased, candid, and educational to the evaluator as well as the court.

As stated above, conducting child custody evaluations arguably may be the most stressful forensic role for a mental health professional. There are many reasons for this perspective. To name but a few: a) the child(ren)'s welfare and well-being are at stake, hinging on decisions about the care, custody, and control of them; b) the fact that a custody evaluation was necessary puts the specific case in a special category, because it means the parties, for probably a myriad of reasons, could not reach a consensus on the custody and child access matters; c) it may mean there are conflicting agendas and goals operating that can consume the litigants, the children, the lawyers, the evaluator, other involved professionals, and the court; d) many of the issues a custody evaluator is asked to address require specialized knowledge, training, and experience; and e) mental health professionals who enter the forensic world of child custody evaluations may do so without fully understanding the nature of the potential adversarial process and what the heat of a litigated custody case may entail.

Striving towards best practices in conducting child custody and child access evaluations is a continual learning process. The reviewer should hope her review testimony and work product, i.e., report, will be a positive learning experience for the evaluator. Unfortunately, our experience is that most evaluators are very defensive in how they respond to the whole idea of being reviewed and sometimes seem to take the review experience as a personal affront. They often tenaciously defend their evaluation and sometimes with charged affect in their testimony under cross-examination. Martindale (2010) made a similar observation and cautioned reviewers to be mindful of the risk management issues involved in doing review work:

> Though many evaluators respond to criticism of their work in a professionally appropriate manner, many others react quite poorly. Of those who react poorly, some appear to have decided that they may be able to intimidate potential critics by filing complaints against those who offer criticism. For that reason, when a forensic psychological consultant comments on the work of a colleague, exposure to risk commences the moment that the reviewer offers the first critical comment . . . Even when complaints are without basis and are quickly dismissed, responding to complaints requires the expenditure of time, energy, and funds (p. 6).

When providing a written report based on a review of a child custody evaluation, we recommend the reviewer include in a section in the report labeled a "caveat on reviewing a colleague's work product." In this section, the reviewer should describe the purpose of a work product review, its limitations, and that the primary goal is to be helpful ("educational") to the court and to the evaluator. As professionals who conduct retained reviews, we genuinely want to educate the evaluator so the evaluator can avoid making similar mistakes in the next custody evaluation. While one of the authors has had the experience of an evaluator deciding never to do another custody evaluation after experiencing a review and hearing rebuttal testimony about the evaluation, this will be the exception. If done well—meaning, in an objective and ethical manner—the the reviewer role can be viewed as part of the process of forensic quality control and an important vehicle to assist the court. The reality is that the court often is not sufficiently aware of or educated about forensic subtleties and specialized knowledge to recognize when the court's appointed expert testimony is inaccurate or misleading. In an ideal sense, reviewers can be viewed as a type of function in the legal process to monitor quality and assess if custody evaluations meet the standards of practice. The reviewer's function may enhance the court's ability to make a thoughtful and educated determination on the issues presented by the custody evaluator's findings and recommendations.

PSYCHOLOGICAL PERSPECTIVE OF THE EVALUATOR
BEING REVIEWED

As noted above, evaluators are often defensive and take opinions in a review as personal criticisms. This may be an understandable human response, but the appropriate professional response is to recognize that retained experts are part of the forensic territory and not uncommon anymore in custody litigation. As mental health professionals who conduct child custody evaluations, we believe we can take some lessons from our legal colleagues, who endure, but (most often) do not personalize criticisms of their reasoning, interpretations, writing, or advocacy. The reviewer is doing his or her job in a legitimate forensic role. Under cross-examination, defensive evaluators may come across as arrogant and cling to flawed data or insufficient methods. Sometimes a reviewer and evaluator will have legitimate differences in professional opinion on a particular issue – methodological preferences for given procedures such as psychological testing, how to interpret or weigh research findings, what is an appropriate parenting time plan for a given age, or how alternative hypotheses were considered. We think it is helpful to the court to hear and weigh these differences.

When significant deficiencies are revealed by a reviewer, and become obvious to the court, then defensiveness by the evaluator will appear to be more ego-protective, or face-saving, rather than the expert evaluator being aligned with the data to be helpful to the court. Sometimes a child custody evaluator who has been reviewed will ask to prepare a rebuttal report to the reviewer's report. Although there is no consensus about whether or not this is an appropriate response, we do think responding to a review via a rebuttal written report runs the risk of the evaluator appearing that he is caught up in a personalized, adversarial stance with the reviewer or with the retaining attorney. As with any expert witness, the evaluator should be mindful of trying to avoid giving "testy" testimony during cross-examination. We strongly recommend the evaluator not write an *ex parte* communication or rebuttal letter to the other counsel (i.e., the one who did not retain the reviewer) or, worse yet, to the court, defending her evaluation.

We recommend that evaluators in every child custody case foresee the possibility of a review and organize her approach to the case with that possibility in mind. This anticipation for the competent evaluator really should not affect the choice of procedures or how thorough the investigation and data collection components are, because those issues should be consistent in each evaluation and conform to practice standards. This anticipation can be helpful to remind evaluators of the importance of keeping a well-organized and legible record or case file that lends itself to an efficient review. The need for keeping a high quality and easy-to-read-and-review file is addressed by

Austin et al. (in press). Our experience is the variance in the quality of record keeping by child custody evaluators is a widespread problem in the field. In most case files that we encounter as reviewers, the handwritten notes are not legible. In such situations the evaluator probably can be required to dictate and have the notes transcribed at his or her own expense. The notes are the core data and if they are not discernible, there is the risk the court may become convinced there are no interview data. Practice guidelines stipulate the need for evaluators to keep a high quality record (APA, 2007) and especially when it is expected there will be a legal proceeding (Specialty Guidelines, 1991).

The psychological posture of the evaluator in response to a review will be enhanced in the eyes of the court if she does not appear defensive and recognizes that the reviewing expert has a legitimate role as part of the legal process. If the evaluator appears to respond to the reviewer's critique and opinions as if they were constructive criticisms, motivated by intended help-fulness, then the evaluator's overall evaluation and opinions may be looked upon more favorably by the court. The court wants to see the evaluator and the reviewer acting in a professional way by being true to the data and issues and providing a thoughtful, thorough, and balanced analysis the court can use in its best interests' analysis.

WORK PRODUCT PRIVILEGE VS. DUTY TO INFORM EVALUATOR

When an individual retains or is appointed an attorney to represent him/her in a legal proceeding, certain privilege rights attach to the attorney-client relationship. If an attorney retains a forensic expert to consult with him or her about the client's case, the privilege extends to the retained psychologist, and the psychologist is prohibited, by law, from contacting anyone or reveal-ing his or her role to anyone, without the attorney's written consent. In con-trast, the APA ethics code (APA, 2002) encourages psychologists to informally resolve situations when it is felt a psychologist may be in violation of the ethics code. The legal and Constitutional protection that is embedded in the attorney-client privilege (*Hickman v. Taylor*, 1947) prevents forensic psy-chologists from adhering to "informal resolutions" in the APA Ethics Code (APA, 2002, 1.04). This prohibition is clearly stated in 1.05 (APA, 2002): "This standard does not apply when an intervention would violate confidentiality rights or when psychologists *have been retained to review the work of another psychologist whose professional conduct is questioned*" [our empha-sis]. This prohibition from making an informal resolution is a professional obligation that applies to the forensic psychologist, as a consulting expert to an attorney, is governed by law and by the rights of the privilege of the attorney's client. Thus, psychologists who expect or demand contact from a colleague when a reviewer finds deficiencies in the custody evaluation are exhibiting a lack of knowledge of the laws of confidentiality and privilege, especially that of attorney-client privilege, and a lack of knowledge of the mandatory limitations on informal attempts at contact between psychologists as spelled out in our Ethics Code (APA, 2002). Unfortunately, our experience is that custody evaluators who have been the subject of a review of their evaluations have made ethical complaints to the American Psychological Association or a state licensing board based on their lack of understanding of the law and a misinterpretation of the ethics code. These ethical complaints against reviewers run the risk of being, in part or whole, perceived as part of the defensive mindset of evaluators when they are reviewed.

The APA Ethics Code (2002) has two primary sections—its General Principles and its Ethical Standards. The five General Principles (Principles A-E) are aspirational in nature. Their goal is "to guide and inspire psychologists towards the very highest ideals of the profession." They are not written as obligations and should not be used to impose sanctions. Pertinent to our discussion here, "[psychologists] are concerned about the ethical compliance of their colleagues' scientific and professional conduct" (APA, 2002, Principle B, Fidelity and Responsibility). Also, "Psychologists exercise reasonable judgment and take precautions to ensure that their potential biases, the boundaries of their competence, and the limitations of their expertise do not lead to or condone unjust practices (APA, 2002, Principle D: Justice). These Principles should guide evaluators and reviewers alike.

The Ethical Standards are not aspirational (APA, 2002). Psychologists who are members of APA are obliged to follow them. These standards are mandatory. Many state licensing boards have adopted in part or whole the APA Ethics Code (CA, FL, NC, PA, SC), so even if a psychologist is not a member of APA, the professional behavior of the licensed psychologist may be governed by the current APA ethics code as it is written into his/her state's licensure law and regulations. In terms of our discussion here, one of the sections of the APA code—Resolving Ethical Complaints—reads "if the conflict between ethics and law, regulations or other governing legal authority" brings the psychologist into a conflict with any of these, the psychologist makes known his/her commitment to the Ethics Code, but if it is unresolvable, after they take steps to resolve it, psychologists "may adhere to the requirements of law, regulations, or other governing legal authority."

Most psychologists learn during their graduate training, that if and when they obtained information that a colleague possibly was exercising questionable ethical judgment or questionable professional behavior, the common ethical rule to consider, if conditions permitted it, was to approach their colleague informally. APA published its first Code of Ethics in 1953 (APA, 1953). The APA has revised its Ethics Code nine times to the current edition adopted by APA in 2002. Consideration of an informal resolution was well established by the eighth revision, Ethical Principles and Code of Conduct by the American Psychological Association (1992): "Psychologists are concerned about the ethical compliance of their colleagues' scientific and professional conduct. When appropriate, they consult with colleagues in order to prevent or avoid unethical conduct" (Principle C: Professional and Scientific Responsibility). Such an informal and diplomatic approach made a lot of sense.

The previous edition of the APA Ethics Code (1992) also had a provision (8.02 Confronting Ethical Issues) encouraging psychologists to consult with other psychologists who are knowledgeable about ethical issues when a psychologist "is uncertain whether a particular situation or course of action would violate this Ethics Code." Further, the previous Code (APA, 1992) had a section (8.04 Informal Resolution of Ethical Violations) that stated, "When psychologists believe that there may have been an ethical violation by another psychologist, they attempt to resolve the issue by bringing it to the attention of that individual *if an informal resolution appears appropriate and the intervention does not violate any confidentiality rights that may be involved*" [emphasis added]. Another section of the 1992 Code (8.05 Reporting Ethical Violations) stated that when an informal resolution intervention did not properly resolve the perceived ethical violation, psychologists were instructed by this Code (APA, 1992) to "take further action appropriate to the situation, *unless such action conflicts with confidentiality rights in ways that cannot be resolved* [emphasis added]. Such action might include referral to state or national committees on professional ethics or to state licensing boards" (p. 1611). As the reader can see, the operant construct—confidentiality—was what psychologists needed to consider prior to initiating an informal intervention. The over-arching concern, it seemed, was psychologists needed to be concerned about what, if any, untoward effects an informal intervention might have on someone's confidentiality rights.

In forensic psychology, as a specialization that attempts to define the intersection between psychology and law, forensic practitioners learn not only what was being alluded to by the term "confidentiality rights," but also whose confidentiality rights needed to be considered. There are often multiple layers of privilege and confidentiality.

There are times (alluded to in the phrase noted above, *if conditions permitted it*), when, in the role of a reviewer, contacting a colleague about his/her questionable professional judgment or behavior, might seem to be desirable, but such contact is not only, itself, unethical, such contact might be illegal and prohibited by law. We have found there is much confusion and disagreement among psychologists about this standard. The previous edition of the APA Ethics Code (1992) alluded to these situations, as noted above, but did not offer much guidance or specificity about informal resolution. The current revision of APA's Ethical Principle and Code of Conduct (2002, 1.04, Informal Resolution of Ethical Violations) more specifically recognizes this limitation, particularly with regard to reviewing the work product of another expert: "When psychologists believe that there may have been an ethical violation by another psychologist, they attempt to resolve the issue by bringing it to the attention of that individual, *if an informal resolution appears appropriate and the intervention does not violate any confidentiality rights that may be involved*" [emphasis added]. The current Ethics Code (APA, 2002, 1.05, Reporting Ethical Violations) states further: "Such action might include referral to state or national committees on professional ethics, to state licensing boards, or to the appropriate institutional authorities. *This standard does not apply when an intervention would violate confidentiality rights or when psychologists have been retained to review the work of another psychologist whose professional conduct is in question*" [emphasis added].

As reviewers, forensic psychologists are engaged ethically and legally as consulting experts to review and critique the work of their colleagues. As stated above, the review work—in its initial phase—comes under the retaining attorney's work product privilege. The review is thus privileged and confidential.

When retained to review someone else's work, under these conditions, as a consulting expert to an attorney, the reviewer is prohibited by law and by her professional ethics from contacting the custody evaluator. The reviewer simply cannot make contact. An informal resolution is prohibited. In the role as a retained reviewer, the reviewer cannot exercise the time-honored practice noted above and memorialized in the Ethical Principles and Code of Conduct (APA, 2002).

It appears that many psychologists still hold the erroneous opinion that contacting a colleague and attempting an informal resolution is a higher ethical standard than adhering to the conduct required of psychologists who are retained as consulting experts by attorneys in civil and criminal law (see Introduction and Applicability, pg. 2, APA, 2002). We believe and understand that it is this misperception among our colleagues about what is *higher* on the legal-moral-ethical continuum that leads to additional conflict and animosity within our profession—most especially when there is a conflict between psychologists in a child custody case who are functioning in a clinical or therapeutic role and those who are functioning in a forensic role.

We are of the opinion that a psychologist cannot and should not expect or demand another psychologist, who has been retained as a confidential consulting expert, and whose work product for that attorney is protected by law under the attorney-client and work product privilege, to agree that the APA Ethics Code (2002) trumps the law and the retained psychologist has an ethical obligation to contact the psychologist to attempt an informal resolution, over and above the legal prohibitions against such contact. The APA (2002, 1.04) ethical code continues to express that a psychologist who believes another psychologist may have violated some professional ethics should consider if a "reasonable resolution appears appropriate," but it also adds that any such intervention must also consider whether or not it violates any confidentiality rights that may be involved" (p. 1063).

In the role of a reviewer, the retained expert has an obligation not to disclose any information until the reviewer-expert is disclosed and identified to be a testifying expert. This prohibition would include even revealing to the evaluator (or anyone, for that matter) the reviewer was a retained expert and was involved in the case at all. There needs to be a shroud of total secrecy until the attorney discloses the existence of the reviewing expert. For the psychologist-reviewer to discuss concerns about the work product with a colleague in an informal way would invite a lawsuit from the attorney or her client, and a legitimate complaint to the reviewer's licensing board and professional organizations for violating confidentiality and privilege.

The ethical tension that exists for psychologists involved in child custody litigation appears (in part) to be caused by friction between the ethical rule on informing colleagues about concerns about their professional conduct versus the preeminent ethical concern for protecting a client's privilege and right of confidentiality. Since the U.S. Supreme Court has addressed and endorsed the sanctity of the confidentiality in the psychologist-client privilege (*Jaffee v. Redmond*, 1996; Shuman & Foote, 1999)—albeit in the context of psychotherapist-client privilege—just as it has regarding the attorney-client privilege (*Hickman v. Taylor*, 1947), it would appear that the ethical and legal duty of privilege and confidentiality trumps the need to inform a colleague about a potential ethical breach. It does not seem like an ethical close call.

The issue of competing demands between professional ethics and law seems to us to be largely a nonissue for several reasons:

1. First, our professional standards direct mental health professionals in the field of child custody evaluation to attempt to resolve such conflicts, but ultimately the professional must make sure his or her behavior comports foremost with the law (AFCC, 2007, Rules P.3, 2.2). The APA Ethics Code (2002) states in Ethical Standard 1.02 Conflicts Between Ethics and Law, Regulations, or Other Governing Legal Authority, "If psychologists' ethical responsibilities conflict with law, regulations, or other governing legal authority, psychologists make known their commitment to the Ethics Code and take steps to resolve it. If the conflict cannot be resolved via such means, psychologists may adhere to the requirements of the law, regulations, or other governing legal authority" (p. 1063).
2. The reviewer and the child custody evaluator need to be mindful of who is the consumer of his or her forensic services. For the evaluator, it is the court. For the reviewer, we would argue, it is the retaining attorney and the court. The retaining attorney is also the advocate for the rights and privileges of his/her client. Thus, the retained consulting expert, when acting in the role of a reviewer, must understand there are two layers of privilege

rights: the one between the attorney and his/her retained expert, and two, the paramount one between the attorney and his/her client.

3. If the psychologist-reviewer finds deficiencies in the methodology and quality of the child custody work product, these deficiencies will not usually rise to a level where there would be an ethical duty to make a report to the APA or to the state licensing board. There is a fundamental distinction between poor quality in the design and implementation of a forensic evaluation and an ethical violation of the APA Ethics Code (2002) or state or provincial licensure regulations, even if the deficiency was sufficient to be considered a fatal flaw so as not to be helpful to the court. If the deficiency was egregious and also an ethical breach of the Code (APA, 2002), then the reviewer would not be free to discuss the matter with the evaluator unless permitted to do so (or released from the privilege of work product privilege) by the retaining attorney. To interpret the APA Ethics Code (2002) as requiring the psychologist-reviewer to discuss the matter with the psychologist-evaluator prior to preparing a review report for the court and testimony is a misinterpretation and misunderstanding of the APA Ethics Code (2002) and pertinent laws regarding confidentiality and privilege.

4. The requirement is to discuss the matter with the psychologist before making an ethical complaint to APA, not before offering a critique, such as an affidavit, or giving testimony in a deposition or in court as an expert witness. Even if a reviewer thinks a complaint should be made to a colleague's ethics board or licensing board, the reviewer cannot do so without permission of the retaining attorney, as the privilege still attaches. For this reason, we think this tension between law and ethics is a nonissue, and does not create an ethical double bind. Courts would not tolerate a requirement by a professional organization to dictate to psychologists that they need to breach attorney-client work product privilege. APA learned long ago that the regulatory power of the federal government supersedes that of a private professional organization (or guild) (APA, 1993).

PRACTICE TIPS: MAKING A CUSTODY EVALUATION REVIEW-PROOF

There is no guarantee a child custody evaluation and written report will not be subject to a work product review. It sometimes will be a favorable review with the expectation that testimony by the reviewer will buttress the evaluator's opinions by attesting to the quality of the work product and that data support the opinions. This favorable testimony by a reviewer might be expected when there were other retained experts (on the other side) who were expected to be critical of the evaluation. There are, however, some basic steps or safeguards for the custody evaluator who wants to have his work product favorably reviewed and received by the court. Every expert wants to be persuasive with the court. Evaluators are advised to consider the following:

1. Conduct self-examination on the depth and breadth of their training in child custody evaluation methodology and knowledge of substantive issues and research, especially on complex and special issues such as domestic violence, intimate partner violence, relocation, child sexual abuse, attachment theory and quality of parent-child relationships, psychological testing, substance abuse, child alienation and estrangement, and cultural issues that might exist.
2. Identify areas of weakness in one's training and experience and be prepared to seek professional consultation in cases for problematic issues.
3. Be fully knowledgeable about professional guidelines and standards for child custody, especially recent publications by AFCC (2007) and APA (2010).
4. Receive training on the literature and research on cognitive biases that often affect custody evaluators.
5. Be vigilant on the consideration of alternative hypotheses that need to be developed and investigated in all custody cases. Confirmatory bias often stems from not considering alternative hypotheses or showing an imbalance in gathering data on important hypotheses on the salient issues.
6. Be knowledgeable about the relevant scientific research literature on issues relevant to each case. Be prepared to "freshen up" on relevant literature when a case begins. Do not make generalized assertions about "the research says," unless you know the research and can cite it. Be sensitive to bias created by a one-sided view of the research literature, e.g., primary caregiver bias, anti-relocation bias, etc.
7. Be knowledgeable about the applicable law for the case. This is one of the greatest weaknesses of custody evaluators. We are not lawyers; but mental health professionals, who are venturing forth into the forensic arena, and need to know the law. To not be adequately informed usually means the correct psycholegal questions will not be asked and data will not be gathered on important factors. Knowing the law is necessary to formulating opinions for the court based on the data.
8. Acknowledge the limitations of the report. Do not avoid concluding that it is not possible to have an opinion for the court in light of the circumstances of the case and the extent of the data. This is a common issue in cases concerning allegations of parental misconduct, e.g., partner violence, child sexual abuse.
9. Make sure all expressed opinions are adequately supported by the data.
10. Be knowledgeable about the principles, research, and application of risk assessment methodology when there are issues of harm involved in the case.

SUMMARY

In this article, we described the evolving role of the reviewer of a colleague's work product in a child custody evaluation context. The standard of practice of the role of a reviewer is developing, as demonstrated by the articles in this special issue of this journal. Ethical and legal issues were discussed, especially the necessary sequence of conducting an objective review of the work product/report before moving towards being designated as a testifying expert or providing forensic consultation services. The article emphasizes that the primary function of the testifying expert/reviewer is to be helpful, not only to the retaining attorney, but to the court. We discussed the challenge for the reviewer to establish credibility with the court in the role of a retained expert. We described the psychological perspective of both reviewer and evaluator and the problem of evaluators being defensive when they are undergoing a review of their professional work product. We examined the issue of the APA ethics code and tradition of psychologists trying to informally resolve ethical concerns. We pointed out that work product and attorney-client privileges would not permit a retained expert to approach a colleague. Colleagues who believe the reviewer should approach them and discuss differences in opinion on the quality of an evaluator's work product are mistaken. There is a clash between law and professional ethics on this issue, but most of the time the deficiencies in the evaluation will not constitute an ethical violation. We discussed how the common practice of reviewers is to combine review work and forensic consultation and how this is compatible with ethical guidelines if there is first an objective review conducted and the reviewer is mindful of giving a balanced and accurate analysis of the evaluator's data and issues, or "impartiality is the best advocacy" (Shuman & Greenberg, 2003, p. 221).

NOTE

1. The Association of Family and Conciliation Courts (AFCC) currently has a task force developing model guidelines for the forensic roles and services of case consultation and work product review.

REFERENCES

Ackerman, M., & Ackerman, M. (1997). Custody evaluation practices: A survey of experienced professionals (Revisited). *Professional Psychology: Research and Practice, 28*, 137–145. doi:10.1037/0735-7028.28.2.137

American Psychological Association (APA). (1953). *Ethical standards for psychologists, Vol. 1, The code of ethics.* Washington, DC: American Psychological Association.

American Psychological Association (APA). (1994). Guidelines for child custody evaluations in divorce proceedings. *American Psychologist, 49*, 677–680. doi:10.1037/0003-066X.49.7.677

American Psychological Association (APA). (1992). Ethical principles of psychologists and code of conduct. *American Psychologist, 47*, 1597–1611. doi:10.1037/0003-066X.47.12.1597

American Psychological Association (APA). (1993, February). Letter to all APA members concerning consent agreement with Federal Trade Commission on restraint of trade, Jack Wiggins, Jr., Ph.D., President.

American Psychological Association (APA). (2002). Ethical principles of psychologists and code of conduct. *American Psychologist, 57*, 1060–1073. doi:10.1037/0003-066X.57.12.1060

American Psychological Association (APA). (2007). Record keeping guidelines. *American Psychologist, 62*(9), 993–1004. doi:10.1037/0003-066X.62.9.993

American Psychological Association (APA). (2010). Guidelines for child custody evaluations in family law proceedings. *American Psychologist, 65*(9), 863–867.

Association of Family and Conciliation Courts (AFCC). (2007). Model standards of practice for child custody evaluation. *Family Court Review, 45*(1), 70–91. doi:10.1111/j.1744-1617.2007.129_3.x

Austin, W. G. (2009). Responding to the call to child custody evaluators to justify the reason for their professional existence: Some thoughts on Kelly and Ramsey (2009). *Family Court Review, 47*(3), 544–551. doi:10.1111/j.1744-1617.2009.01272.x

Austin, W. G., Dale, M. D., Kirkpatrick, H. D., & Flens, J. R. (2011). Forensic expert roles and services in child custody litigation: Work product review and case consultation. *Journal of Child Custody, 8*(1/2), 47–83.

Austin, W. G., Kirkpatrick, H. D., & Flens, J. R. (2011). The emerging forensic role of work product review and case analysis in child access and parenting plan disputes. *Family Court Review, 49*(4).

Bow, J. N., & Boxer, P. (2003). Assessing allegations of domestic violence in child custody evaluations. *Journal of Interpersonal Violence, 18*(12), 1394–1410. doi:10.1177/0886260503258031

Bow, J. N., & Quinnell, F. A. (2001). Psychologists' current practices and procedures in child custody evaluations: Five years post American Psychological Association guidelines. *Professional Psychology: Research and Practice, 32*, 261–268. doi:10.1037/0735-7028.32.3.261

Bow, J. N., & Quinnell, F. A. (2002). A critical review of child custody evaluation reports. *Family Court Review, 40*(2), 164–176. doi:10.1111/j.174-1617.2002.tb00827.x

Bow, J. N., & Quinnell, F. A. (2004). Critique of child custody evaluations by the legal profession. *Family Court Review, 42*, 115–127.

Committee on Ethical Guidelines for Forensic Psychologists (1991). Specialty guidelines for forensic psychologists. *Law and Human Behavior, 15*, 655–665. doi:10.1007/BF01065858

Gould, J. W., Kirkpatrick, H. D., Austin, W. G., & Martindale, D. (2004). A framework and protocol for providing a forensic work product review: Application to child custody evaluations. *Journal of Child Custody: Research, Issues, and Practices, 1*(3), 37–64. doi:10.1300/J190v01n03_04

Heilbrun, K. (2001). *Principles of forensic mental health assessment.* New York: Kluwer Academic/Plenum Publishers.

Hickman v. Taylor, 329 U.S. 495 (1947).

Horvath, L. S., Logan, T. K., & Walker, R. (2002). Child custody cases: A content analysis of evaluations in practice. *Professional Psychology: Research and Practice, 33*, 557–565. doi:10.1037/0735-7028.33.6.557

Jaffee v. Redmond, 518 U.S. 1 (1996).

Kelly, R. F., & Ramsey, S. H. (2009). Child custody guidelines: The need for systems-level outcome assessments. *Family Court Review, 47*(2), 286–303. doi:10.1111/j.1744-1617.2009.01255.x

Kirkpatrick, H. D. (2004). A floor, not a ceiling: Beyond guidelines—An argument for minimum standards of practice in conducting child custody and visitation evaluations. *Journal of Child Custody: Research, Issues, and Practices, 1*, 61–76. doi:10.1300/J190v01n01_05

Martindale, D. A. (2010). Psychological experts and trial tactics: The impact of unarticulated contingencies. *The Matrimonial Strategist, 28*(8), 5–6.

Martindale, D. A., & Gould, J. W. (2008). Evaluating the evaluators in custodial placement disputes. In H. Hall (Ed.) *Forensic psychology and neuropsychology for criminal and civil cases* (pp. 527–546; 923–935). Boca Raton, FL: Taylor & Francis.

Mnookin, J. L., & Gross, S. R. (2003). Expert information and expert testimony: A preliminary taxonomy. *Seton Hall Law Review, 34*, 139–185.

Shuman, D. W., & Foote, W. (1999). Jaffee v. Redmond's impact: Life after the Supreme Court's recognition of a psychotherapist-patient privilege. *Professional Psychology: Research and Practice, 30*(5), 479–487. doi:10.1037/0735-7028.30.5.479

Shuman, D. W., & Greenberg, S. A. (2003). The expert witness, the adversary system, and the voice of reason: Reconciling impartiality and advocacy. *Professional Psychology: Research and Practice, 34*(3), 219–224. doi:10.1037/0735-7028.34.3.219

Stahl, P. (1996). Second opinions: An ethical and professional process for reviewing child custody evaluations. *Family and Conciliation Courts Review, 34*, 386–395. doi:10.1111/j.174-1617.1996.tb00428.x

Tippins, T. M. (2009). Expert witnesses and consultants. *The Matrimonial Strategist, 27*(3), 1, 3–4.

Commentary on Forensic Mental Health Consulting: Is More Better?

MARK JUHAS

Superior Court of California, Los Angeles, California

Family law in the twenty first century is rapidly changing; included in that change is the once predictable role of the mental health professional. Increasingly, the court relies on the professional to help explain to both the court and the parties the details of the parenting plans that are proposed. This article suggests that a retained mental health evaluator has a much greater role to play in resolution of the case, thus helping the dissolving family to a mutual resolution, rather than ongoing litigation. The mental health professional can also assist the court in determining what parenting plan is best for the family by clarifying the various recommendations for both the court and the parties. Finally, the mental health evaluator can be very helpful to the court in sitting down with the parties and addressing some of the families concerns with the evaluator's recommendations. The mental health evaluator can then assist the litigants in a facilitative way to structure plans that are truly in the best interest of the family.

Every day across the country, in both formal evidentiary hearings and less formal motions and orders to show cause, families ask judicial officers to make decisions, which will define the future course of the entire family for years to come.

Because parents must come to court for custody and visitation orders, court users represent a broad array of individuals, each of whom want essentially the same thing: some order in their lives. Many of these cases involve professionals such as attorneys and child custody evaluators, but some do not. In my courtroom family law attorneys are becoming increasingly rare; upwards of 70% of the litigants are self-represented. In domestic violence cases, the self-represented can climb to a staggering 90% or more. Other professionals in the family law system may or may not see this depending on the nature of their practice and geographic location, but this circumstance has drastically changed the way the family court functions.

Many litigants—both represented and unrepresented—come into the court with unrealistic expectations about possible outcomes of the litigation and no meaningful understanding of the limitations on those results. Most litigants simply do not understand that in family court the vast majority of the parents are good enough and the bench officer will recognize this fact. Many of those who choose to self-represent manage the court process very well. But, the majority struggle with the court's evidentiary and procedural requirements. The court increasingly finds itself in the unenviable position of having to make significant life altering decisions for a family on scant information with parties that are manifestly unfamiliar with how to respond to the law's requirements.

It is also no secret that family law courts nationwide are under resourced. This includes not only insufficient numbers of bench officers, but also limits on the programs that the court is either statutorily required to provide or that the court determines are essential to its function. This lack of adequate court resourcing manifests itself through impossibly long courtroom calendars, seemingly endless lines at clerk windows, over stressed self-help centers, and long wait times for mediation appointments, to name but a few. All of this adds up to a family law system that is bursting at the seams and often has an insufficient ability to provide each family the time it needs to have its concerns fully addressed.

In most jurisdictions, as it is in my courtroom, family law courts are full-service for the litigants, meaning that the court is not specifically trained or tasked to handle only one type of case, such as custody or property. On my typical Order to Show Cause (OSC) calendar for example, there may be custody requests, property disputes, discovery motions, free-standing domestic violence restraining orders and requests for child and spousal support, and so forth, all to be handled in the space of a few hours. Each of these also has a different statutory priority making any given case more or less urgent relative to the other matters on the calendar. Adding to the confusion is the fact that my courtroom is not designated to handle specific types of cases based on their size or complexity, unlike most civil courtrooms. My calendar each day depends on who got to the courthouse when, and what they need addressed. The first matter on calendar may involve a marital estate of substantial size with concurrent high incomes and children, while the next case may very well involve a family with no children and only debt to their name as both parties were recently laid off. Both cases are equally important and, frankly, may absorb an equivalent amount of bench time.

The aforementioned concerns are then coupled with the fact that both the law itself and the dissolution process are complex, time consuming, and often confusing to the most seasoned family law attorney, let alone those who chose to self-represent. It is easy for those of us who toil every day in family law to lose sight of the complexity of the law as well as misperceive the difficulty of the dissolution process; both the law and the process become more time intensive with each passing year, there are new statutory requirements, new and modified forms, and new procedural courtroom obligations. Additionally, in Southern California, as in other parts of the country, litigants frequently suffer from cultural and language barriers. Litigants with limited English proficiency are at an even greater disadvantage in the system; not only do they not understand the language, but depending on where in the world they call home, they may not even trust the legal system. Because the bench officer may be the only legal expert in the hearing, these factors also add to the time stress and obligations of the bench officer.

As should be clear from this backdrop, the modern family law courtroom is a busy, somewhat frantic, and under-resourced place. While the vast majority of the court's work is done outside of the courtroom, what happens in the courtroom often is the focus for many litigants. Many families want the court's attention and there are precious few hours in the day to provide access to a bench officer. The courtroom is a zero-sum game; every minute taken up by one family is taken away from another. While family law bench officers attempt, as much as possible, to maximize the time on the bench, they cannot do it alone. Increasingly, bench officers seek ways to streamline cases by reducing or eliminating irrelevant or marginally useful information and requiring more settlement efforts. Experts are part of this as well; bench officers look to both neutral experts as well as retained experts to provide insightful information as well as help the parties better understand the needs of the children. Judicial officers have become far more diligent in precluding or limiting experts that have little value or are insufficiently prepared. Courts no longer have the luxury of listening to long, rambling presentations of facts or opinions that have very little bearing on the family at bar. It is critical that the expert, attorney, and litigant understand and are respectful of the time pressures that the bench officer faces.

Courts also recognize that investing the parties with the ability to make the decisions themselves is often a far superior method of case resolution than is forcing them into a litigation path. All too often both the children and the fact that most families have finite financial resources gets lost in the litigation; all too often the litigation takes on a life of its own, not ending until one or both of the parties are financially impoverished or have a broken spirit. Far too frequently, not only the family, but the experts and attorneys (and perhaps even the court) lose sight of the fact that the goal of family law is to transition the family from one configuration to another, not to destroy the family's very fabric. After the case is finished, the parents must still raise the child to be a responsible adult; if the litigation process destroys the parents' ability to meaningfully co-parent, then the system tragically fails the parents and their children.

Because of the crush of litigation and a recognition of the toll on the family, the court is, with greater frequency, requiring the parties to make good faith attempts to resolve the matter on their own and the court is looking to other professionals for help in this process. In many courts mental health experts (as well as other professionals) have proven invaluable in early intervention case resolution conferences shortly after a case was filed, but before litigation starts in earnest. These experts can sit and talk to the parents and perhaps even the children if appropriate, helping the family resolve the matter on their own. These experts find themselves in a very unique position early in the case, before positions are hardened by pride or litigation. They educate the parents about not only the needs of the children, but the child custody process itself. Armed with this helpful information, many parties will determine that it is best to resolve the matter informally rather than through hard fought litigation in court. Such an informal resolution may very well cause the family to proceed with success rather than the failure of litigation-induced self destruction.

Traditionally, the mental health professional had a limited and clearly defined role. The parties would ask the court to hire a neutral evaluator expert who had one job and one job only—to fully evaluate the family, provide a written report to the court and testify if needed. In light of the shifting needs of the court and the parties, the roles of experts have changed and expanded beyond this traditional approach. Currently, courts are asking and expecting experts to do their work with an eye toward resolution of the case as well as educating both the bench and the litigants on many different facets of the family. These new roles can be invaluable to the family law process but each is fraught with ethical and professional challenges.

With increasing frequency, if an early settlement is not possible, a neutral expert may be brought into a case and find that one or both sides are not represented. The neutral expert's "job description" vis-à-vis the court may be very different if one or both of the parties do not have attorneys. Depending on the case and the affluence of the parties, this expert may be the only professional working with the parties. If the court provides only broad and somewhat vague instructions and guidance, the expert may very well feel somewhat at loose ends. In the case of self-represented litigants, they may have vastly different agendas from each other both of which are at odds with the court's needs. These cases can prove to be challenging as the neutral expert is almost certainly the only one who knows what the judge needs in order to make orders and may feel compelled to guide the evaluation or even make some tactical decisions along the way. Nevertheless, this expert is able to talk to the parties and describe for them what he is seeing in the family. This is an opportunity for the expert to teach the parent what he knows about and what he is finding in the family. If presented correctly, this information may have the effect of allowing the parents to pull together for their children, as opposed to becoming further polarized.

The neutral evaluator is in a unique position to either help guide the family through the process to a mutually satisfactory resolution, or guide the family directly into the courthouse depending on how they approach their task. Litigation is rarely as cathartic or one sided as the parties might hope because the court infrequently vindicates one side at the expense of the other. To be sure, an evaluator cannot ethically step outside of his role, but an evaluator can certainly talk to the family about the challenges of litigating the case. While the evaluator can and should rigorously protect and foster his neutrality, at the same time he can and should use the evaluation as a teaching and learning process for the parents so that they are given more than cold opinions and recommendations. Part of the expert's goals should be to give the family the opportunity to develop the tools needed to successfully move into the future. One of these tools clearly is the ability to compromise for the children's greater good.

From the beginning of the expert's involvement in the case, the expert's relationship with the family can be challenging for both the expert and the family. In highly contested cases, the parties will try to gain a litigation advantage at every turn in the proceedings. It is critical to the process that the expert be viewed as neutral and above reproach. If either side loses confidence in the manner that the case is being handled, this not only undermines the expert's opinions, but it may cause the family great emotional stress and financial loss. If the expert becomes a distraction in the litigation, the focus in the case may shift from the children and the family to the needs of the expert, the legal professionals, and the very litigation itself. Once the expert becomes the issue in the case, the parties undoubtedly begin to harbor concerns as to the expert's neutrality, thus hampering the expert's ability to evaluate and assist the family; this needlessly drags out the litigation. Many times it is the constant friction around unresolved parenting time issues that leads to very poor outcomes for the family in litigation.

If the expert allows him or her self to be dragged into the litigation fray, it may appear to both the court and the parties that the expert has stepped outside of a neutral role. The purpose of an evaluation is to establish a workable and appropriate parenting plan for the child in the case. At the end of the process, the parties need and want an order that they can and will follow. They did not come to court for anything less; if we do not deliver that outcome we have left the family worse off than we found it, with less money, greater distrust, and still no workable solution for the child. In an extreme case where the expert is a constant source of dispute the court may have no choice but to relieve the expert and start all over, or proceed without an expert. Either way the family loses, as there is now delay and increased confusion in the litigation.

Having said all of this, the neutral custody evaluator remains a critical part of the process for many parents. The expert brings a certain amount of dispassionate expertise to the family. This expert, more than anyone else in the case has the unique ability to talk with all of the parties. Because the evaluator does not "choose sides," he or she has the ability to point out to both parents those things that they do well as parents, as well as those parenting areas that need improvement. In those cases that present significant conflict, the expert can take a view from a distance and suggest parenting classes, counseling, and a wide range of tools that give the parents the opportunity to stop the warfare and focus on their children. Of course, it is up to the individuals involved to stop what they are doing, but the evaluator is often the only individual with both the knowledge and the credibility to make the parties consider other alternatives to the ongoing conflict that is so destructive for the children. Additionally, the expert has the ability to consensus build between the parties to move toward a parenting plan that makes sense for the family.

The same economic pressures that limit court budgets today also impact family finances. The family may simply not have the economic wherewithal to pay the cost of a full child custody evaluation requiring the expert to perform a limited scope evaluation. While this does not change the complexity of the issues before the court, it does challenge the evaluator to assist the family on a shoe-string. In some ways, the limited scope evaluation brings into even greater focus the landmines for the expert, as the expert is attempting to make do with less information and time. Many evaluators are becoming quite adept at providing limited-scope evaluations with limited expenditure of resources. While the expert finds himself in the position of making decisions based solely on the economics of the family, the expert can provide a real service to the court and the family by making recommendations and suggesting resolution on a shortened time schedule. Such an evaluation makes available to a greater number of people certain expertise on family issues. Again, this gives the family greater information upon which to base decisions about the future.

Many neutral evaluators, both full and limited scope, are currently sitting down with the parties at an informal feedback session either before or after the report is written, or even in lieu of the report, wherein the expert's opinions are discussed at length among the parties. Not only does this help the parties reach a resolution, but it also allows them the advantage of the expert's thought process before the matter proceeds to trial. Many times this feedback session allows the parties to review their positions, contemplate the recommendations and the evaluator's comments, and reach an agreement on the case. These sessions allow the expert and the parties to fine tune the facts and make sure that the expert "got it right" from the parties perspective. From the court's perspective, these feedback sessions allow the parties a good opportunity to determine their own future and settle the case if they wish to do so. Further, it also saves court time as it forces the parties to focus their thoughts thus making for better and streamlined presentations.

If the evaluator expert writes a report, this report must clearly and concisely set forth the facts that the expert relied on as well as fully fleshing out the reasons for the conclusions reached. The report must be grounded in the research and the literature so that the parties are given the opportunity to know how the opinions were reached. Sadly, many child custody evaluations are long on family history and short on the unique aspects of each parent that make the specific parent/child relationship work well or not work at all. It is this detail that allows the court to have a better insight into the family and provides greater support for the ultimate orders. It is this detail that sheds light on the family and its attributes, which allows the court to fashion meaningful and appropriate orders. It is this detail that educates and enlightens the family itself. Such a recitation of the facts and the resulting recommendations gives the family a structure within which to meaningfully discuss resolution of the case short of all out litigation.

Once the court has ordered a child custody evaluation and the report is issued, one party may simply take issue with the report's expressed opinions. Or conversely, the evaluator's recommendations and comments may very well miss the mark for this family because of many different factors. The evaluator may have misapplied the developmental theory, misunderstood the facts or the culture of the family, or maybe even simply got it wrong. In order to proffer an alternate parenting plan, or attack the evaluator's proposals, the "out" parent must get reliable and admissible evidence before the court. The only real way to do this is through an additional retained expert. Depending on how this expert is hired and what the expert is trying to accomplish, this expert may be of little or great value to the court.

Emotions often run high in a litigated custody matter. In family law, many times parents take a very black and white view of the world; individuals, including professionals in the litigation, are either with them or against them. If the neutral evaluator takes a position that is adverse to a party, frequently that party will summarily dismiss the opinion, even though it is the right result for this family. A party's own expert may be able to take some of the sting out of the adverse opinions allowing for a less emotionally-laden view of the case. This is especially true, as the party's own expert may be viewed as being aligned with that party thus having more credibility. If this discussion avoids a lengthy, expensive, and highly conflicted trial, this is obviously good for the parties. In the appropriate case, this "voice of reason" would allow the party a comfortable way to resolve the matter short of a trial.

Additionally, the retained expert can work with the party's attorney and educate the legal professional as to the correctness of the neutral's recommendations. The attorney may have misunderstood or misperceived the actual facts of the case, the family's needs, or the thrust of the recommendations. Not only is the expert in a position to aid the attorney in preparing for court, the expert may be able to better advise the attorney of the likely outcome of the matter should it be tried. Such a dialogue between the attorney and the expert may very well avoid an unnecessary trial of the case.

If the neutral evaluator misperceived the needs of the family, the party may retain an expert to challenge the evaluator's opinions. Sometimes the evaluator does not fully understand the families' culture or misperceives some other factual basis in the evaluation. Or, the evaluator may have gone down some superficially appealing path that simply will not withstand scrutiny. Because the party's independently retained expert will likely not have access to the children, the other party and many of the collaterals that the court's expert interviewed, the opinions of this expert will likely be severely limited in court. What this expert can do is gather the cultural or other factual errors together as well as the scientific errors and present them to the court, thus aiding the bench officer in making the orders. Further, a discussion between this expert and the other side may very well enlighten the opposition that there are fatal flaws in the evaluation that render it of limited value.

If the evaluator failed to take into consideration the current literature as part of the evaluation or misapplied it to the current family, a separately retained expert may have great value to the court. While there are numerous educational opportunities for bench officers, bench officers simply do not have time to read and digest all of the current literature to keep up with the latest thinking of mental health professionals in the area of family law. In the right case, it would be extremely helpful to the bench to have a well-organized presentation that presents a useful, but accurate, overview of the current thought in the main child development issues before the court. Bench officers are like all other adult learners: some are visual, some are auditory, but all are time stressed. If the expert could put together a concise presentation on the issue in the case as well as a brief overview of the literature with a few clean, simple and engaging visual aids (even PowerPoint) this may very well cause the court to reconsider the recommendations. Such a presentation would be welcome in either a settlement or setting or a full blown evidentiary hearing. Aside from challenging the neutral evaluation in court, one party may retain a mental health professional to assist that party in the preparation and presentation of the case. These experts provide great service to the parties by helping them prepare for the litigation and to better understand the needs of the children and the various strengths and weaknesses of the family structure. This expert could prove to play an invaluable role in the case. This expert provides the party with a strong understanding of the literature and an expert review of the report, from a factual and philosophical point of view. If the party is well prepared and able to fully understand the neutral's opinions, the party is far more likely to have a concise and meaningful presentation to the bench officer. Additionally, such an expert will be able to assist the party in challenging the other side's presentation. This type of presentation and preparation increases the ability of the bench officer to fully understand the case and the various needs of the family.

Of all of the ways to use a retained expert, the least useful is to challenge the methodology of the report. It is critically important that any expert follow the guidelines and the rules of the profession. This is especially true in the family law arena as there are few hard and fast rules and obligations because each family and its situation are different. Plainly, the expert must follow the appropriate protocols in rendering his opinions and must certainly demonstrate that the opinion reached is not merely his subjective view. Nevertheless, if all the party's expert can offer is a critique of the method of the report, the party proposing that expert should think long and hard before presenting the evidence. Often the detailed testimony of rule breaking may be exceptionally important in a purely intellectual setting, but equally true is the fact that it may have little real practical value to the judge's decision-making process. This type of testimony is generally time-consuming and confusing, rendering it hard to follow; there is a risk that the judge will simply discount it all. By placing unnecessary time pressure on the court, the proffering party may very well take time away from far more important and fruitful evidence and testimony.

Further, this type of testimony is often of limited usefulness because a court is ethically bound to determine a case on its merits. The bench officer is more likely focused on the witnesses that testify in the courtroom and factual assertions that go to the merits of the dispute. While the custody evaluation may be the main focus between the experts, to the bench officer it is one piece of evidence to consider in rendering a ruling. Frequently, there is not a nexus between the alleged rule breaking and whether there would have been a difference in the underlying opinion. The court would focus more on the merits of the parties' presentation and the expert's credibility in rendering any decision. Unless the evaluator has simply not followed the professional guidelines in such an obvious manner rendering the opinions truly suspect, the bench officer will no doubt discount this testimony. From a very practical and real standpoint, an expert does great damage to the family and wastes a great deal of time if they inappropriately embolden a party to continue with litigation based on the thin reed of challenging the methodology of the evaluation, unless the challenge is quite compelling.

Another area that an un-retained, neutral expert has great value is as a mediator or a settlement officer in a high conflict case after the evaluation has been conducted. Several courts have used volunteer mental health professionals to great advantage to sit and talk to litigants about their family. Solutions to some of the issues that divorcing families face are counterintuitive, but once an uninvolved qualified individual explains them to the family, this may allow warring parents to understand the value in the proposed plan.

Mental health professionals have a wealth of experience that they bring to a settlement conference that is different from retired judges or practicing attorneys. If the parties have lost confidence in the evaluator, or are simply intractable, a seasoned independent mental health professional may be able to break the stalemate. Unlike the evaluator who may feel compelled to defend the recommendations or the methodology of the report, this new set of eyes has the ability to talk through the fears and concerns of the parties after the evaluation has been performed. With proper facilitation, the parties may be willing to talk, become less invested in their position, and be far more interested in reaching consensus rather than keeping the fight alive. Further, if a judge or legal professional is to participate in the settlement conference, having a neutral mental health professional present may very well allow the discussion between the parties to focus more on the children, rather than focusing on the minutiae of the various recommendations.

Many litigants (both represented and self represented) fear that the court will simply read and then "rubber stamp" the expert's parenting plan. Having a mental health professional present in the conference may very well allay those fears. This individual can allow the parties the opportunity to fully discuss the recommendations and determine whether a few modifications are truly in order. Allowing the parties the opportunity to talk about the report, to dissect it, and to consider it with a trained professional may not cause the case to resolve. But after such a session the parties more likely better understand the recommendations and may not feel like the bench officer imposed those recommendations without a meaningful opportunity to be heard. Again, this type of discussion also gives the parties a chance to focus their concerns, which will make them better able to communicate them to the bench officer. Whether represented or not, if the litigants walk out of the courtroom feeling that they had a significant say in the process, they are more likely to comply with the orders. The expert has a great potential for assisting both the court and the litigants in this setting.

Getting a case to judgment in the twenty-first century family court can be challenging. Parties may take several days off work and sit for hours in a packed courtroom to have the bench officer spend precious little time with them. Many litigants tire of the constant expenditure of their assets for collateral services such as child custody evaluations, minor's counsel, and parenting coordinators for which they perceive little value. Courts, lawyers, and experts need to be mindful of the intrusion and expense that each of these various disciplines bring to the family. Increasingly, one or both of the parents in a custody case may not be represented or may be represented by counsel that is not fully conversant with family law. It is within in this context that a qualified expert retained by one or both of the parties can assist not only the court, but also the parents.

Modern family law could not function without the help of knowledgeable and dedicated mental health professionals; without their able assistance, the outcomes for families would likely be far different. The role of all participants in family law is rapidly changing and the pace of change will only increase. The pace and nature of these changes place mental health professionals squarely in a position to be flexible in their approach and guide families toward resolution and away from needless litigation.

A View from the Cross-Road: Considerations for Mental Health Professionals Consulting with Attorneys (by a Judge, and Former Lawyer ... with a Degree in Psychology)

DIANNA GOULD-SALTMAN

Superior Court of California, Los Angeles, California

In reviewing the articles published in this issue, I find a need to step back to get a perspective on the populations from which each constituency (judges, mental health professionals, attorneys, and parents) views the issue of mental health professionals consulting with attorneys in the context of child custody cases. My own perspective is that of a relatively newly-appointed judge who has practiced family law for 25 years. To some extent, when addressing this issue from the authors' own unique perspectives, there is a bit of Rashomon[1] at work.

From the perspective of the Court, judicial officers see a wide variety of cases. In many jurisdictions a majority of parents appear unrepresented by counsel. Those without attorneys may not have a strong understanding of how the court system works and how decisions about child custody are made. They may be in court addressing child custody, not because their issues are severe or that the disputes are highly contested, but just because they do not know how otherwise to formally resolve child custody issues in any way other than to "go to court." Judicial officers also see well-financed, high-conflict custody cases that may be litigated to the fullest extent the parties can afford. Those parties may or may not have exhausted other possibilities for resolving their child-custody related disputes outside the courtroom setting. Often the judicial officers will see contested custody cases, which have significant complexity and sufficiently high conflict, but where the parties simply lack the financial resources (or time, or advice) to appropriately address the presenting issues. This is a family court judge's universe.

Importantly, and relevant to the subject of this issue, family law judicial officers do not have a homogeneous view of their role in a child custody case. Some view family law as a subset of civil law (which, technically, it is) and treat family law cases as they would other civil cases, albeit aware of the heightened emotions that often accompany family law litigation. And, family law judicial officers realize that, unlike most other civil cases, a ruling in family law involving children is rarely the end of the litigants' relationship to each other. Nevertheless, judges who take this position view their role as decision-maker. A question is submitted to them by the parties and they provide an answer. Other judicial officers see their role as far different from other civil judges. They believe that their obligation is to the children and view their role as a hybrid of decision-maker-social worker (and, in some cases, super-parent). Judicial officers who have this view of their role may employ various means of protecting children within their orders such as appointing parenting plan coordinators to oversee conflict resolution on an ongoing basis. They might also appoint counsel for the child (or guardians ad litem, depending on the jurisdiction) to check in with the family, with the authority to independently institute proceedings on the child's behalf as necessary, and set review hearings in the court, itself.

Attorneys see a different slice of life. Even attorneys whose practice is exclusively family law usually have a fair number of cases that do not involve child custody at all. Where there are minor children, even as some attorneys may consult with parents who cannot afford to hire them, and some may take on pro bono cases. For the most part, the attorney's world is populated by parents who can afford to hire attorneys (or at least have access to other people's money to do so). In the world of most attorneys who deal with child custody, most of those cases will settle through some form of negotiation on a long-term basis without going to court. Only a small portion will require an evaluation. Most of those will resolve without going to court, or without going to court on all issues. So, if only some cases involve children, and those cases can afford attorneys, and most will not require evaluations and most of those which do involve evaluations will settle without going to court, it is only that small slice of the remainder that forms the confluence between the attorney's universe and that of the judge.

The forensic mental health professional's universe is even more rarified. Excluding for the moment forensic mental health professionals (FMHP) who conduct evaluations (which is a separate topic for a different day), those FMHPs who work in a reviewing or consulting role with attorneys are working in a very small subset of child custody litigation. These cases are sufficiently funded to afford both an evaluation and consultants, whether or not they ultimately serve in a testimonial or non-testimonial capacity.

From a parent-litigant's perspective, a FMHP has one of two broad roles. The FMHP may be part of the litigation team with the attorneys (much as a paralegal, accountant, or other expert would be). Alternatively, the FMHP is working directly with the parent-litigant to prepare the parent-litigant for the evaluation process, educate the parent-litigant about parenting issues, psychological literature, or reduce the parent-litigant's anxiety about the process by explaining the process in terms the parent-litigant can understand and manage. FMHPs who work directly with parent-litigants may be seen by the parent-litigant, at times, to be serving a role which, from a lay perspective, may be difficult to distinguish from a therapeutic role. While the professional may understand and intend the relationship to be quite different from a therapeutic one, the parent-litigant who used to feel anxious and upset and who has been calmed down about the process by a "therapist," may see that difference as semantic.

From these three vantage points (judge, attorney, parent-litigant), I consider some of the roles of a consultant discussed in the articles in this issue. As mentioned herein, generally accepted testifying FMHP roles as including, "(1) court appointed, neutral evaluator; (2) case-blind didactic expert, who only provides information about research without having reviewed any case related documents; (3) testifying, evaluating expert hired by one side to conduct an evaluation; and (4) work product reviewer, hired by one side, who, after having completed a review, testifies to his/her assessment of the work reviewed." Let me take each role from each of the three perspectives.

Court-Appointed Neutral Evaluator

The court-appointed, neutral evaluator's value to the Court, to whom the evaluator owes his or her ultimate allegiance, is precisely that singular, neutral role. The Court is likely to receive plenty of non-neutral evidence and testimony, but the Court's ability to rely on the neutrality of the appointed evaluator is the foundation for the appointment. That neutrality works, in part, because there is a "buy-in" by the parties and the attorneys. Only with the assurance that the evaluator starts out neutral and will remain neutral (while gathering data before forming opinions), will the parties and other witnesses be comfortable sharing important information with that evaluator.

Some attorneys and parents may believe that there is a benefit to using an evaluator with a known bias on an issue which favors that party (pro-mothers, pro-father, bias against overnights for young children, etc.). It has been my experience that there is little value to that. The stronger the evaluator's bias, the easier it is to uncover and the court is likely to find any opinions or recommendations of that evaluator less valuable. As a settlement tool, a blatantly lopsided evaluation leaves little room for negotiation. Alternatively, a neutral evaluator who identifies parenting strengths and weaknesses with sufficient data to back up any conclusions will be useful to a Court (should the matter be litigated) and to the parents by providing the basis for settlement, by identifying areas of parenting strength (which can allay concerns of the other parent) and areas needing improvement.

While identified parenting weaknesses are sometimes used as fodder for attack by the other parent, they can also be used by the parent so identified as an opportunity to show the Court that he or she "heard" what the evaluator had to say and jumped in to begin improving his or her parenting.

Case-Blind Didactic Expert

The case-blind didactic testifying expert may be helpful in a limited capacity, if the issues are unique or the judicial officer is relatively new to family law. This should be the case because, ideally, an expert should only be appointed when expertise is necessary: if common knowledge on an issue would suffice, there is no legal basis on which to appoint an expert. For example, most judges would know that, absent issues of violence or substance abuse, young children benefit from the participation of both parents. It is probably not necessary to have a mental health professional testify about that or the literature that supports that. If there is something unique that makes participation of both parents inadvisable in a particular case, this would be unusual and might be something that testimony of a mental health professional would assist the judge to understand.

Some attorneys use a didactic expert to explain issues that are (or should be) a matter of common knowledge. Those attorneys run a risk of over-complicating a case unnecessarily. Those who use such experts to try to create the impression that a psychological issue is "well-decided" in a singular direction run an additional risk: good attorneys on cross-examination will disclose that there are few issues on which there is unanimity in the psychological community. Those who would testify that there is unanimity will be viewed as citing lopsided literature to bolster the position they are being paid to support. Parent-litigants may believe their case is benefitted by hiring a FMHP who will testify based on limited or one-sided presentation of the literature that supports their position. It is the job of the attorney to explain to the parent-litigant how this reduces credibility, which could ultimately affect the outcome of the case.

The One-Sided Evaluator

The testifying evaluator hired by one side to conduct an evaluation is unusual (except in jurisdictions where each side is expected to hire a separate expert and parallel evaluations are conducted simultaneously). Other than in that exceptional case, the one-sided evaluator conducting either a simultaneous evaluation or a subsequent evaluation after the conclusion of a court-appointed evaluation, will always have a different set of data than the first evaluator. The participants' perception of that second evaluator is likely to affect the extent to which the participants will be willing to disclose information and it is that interview information which does, and should, form a significant part of the basis for any conclusions drawn by the evaluator. A one-sided evaluator who has access to only one parent may not have sufficient data to form any opinion about an appropriate parenting arrangement. Those who fail to refrain from opining on that which exceeds their data may actually hinder the Court's work and harm the case for the attorneys who hire them.

From Court's perspective, in my experience, the information provided by a one-sided evaluator is given very little weight. The exception may be when the evaluator is hired to focus on a limited issue and so would not need full information that a custody evaluator would need (e.g., a mental status examination of one parent to determine whether that parent understands the proceedings).

The Work-Product Reviewer

The work-product reviewer who testifies regarding the methodology of the underlying evaluation may be useful by assisting the Court in drawing the boundaries of the same evaluation. Especially when courts have limited resources and where members of the family law bench are new to family law, the work-product reviewer may be the only check and balance for a substandard evaluation, other than cross-examination. A newer judge might not know the extent to which it is inappropriate to draw broad conclusions from very limited data or fail to entertain multiple hypotheses regarding what is going on in a family and only seek data that support a hypothesis developed early in the evaluation process. A work-product reviewer could identify, not just where the data might have led to a different recommendation, but circumstances where the Court should not rely on the data gathered, even if the recommendations are discarded.

Assuming for the moment that this reviewer is ethical and would not testify that an evaluation report which is, overall, supported by appropriate data is not sound, a reviewer may direct the Court to significant flaws in the evaluator's methodology, or the evaluator's analysis. The reviewer also might direct the Court's attention to the absence of a professional nexus between the data, the analysis and the conclusions and recommendations, which go beyond the evaluator's expertise. A reviewer falls short when he or she (a) attempts to decimate an evaluation report without offering any alternatives to throwing everything out and starting fresh or (b) makes recommendations for custody without having better, more or different data than the original evaluator had (and if the reviewer does have such data, he or she is no longer a reviewer: now he or she is just another evaluator with a different opinion).

From the perspective of the attorney, a work-product reviewer, in addition to assisting in the courtroom, may be able to explain to the attorney, and help the attorney explain to the parent-litigant, the strengths and weaknesses of the report, advise regarding implementation of recommendations in the report, and let the attorney and the parent-litigant know "when to fold 'em," in terms of trying to attack good work. In this sense, all work-product reviewers necessarily start as a non-testifying consultant. Only those who would offer to testify against an evaluation report sight unseen would do otherwise. If the underlying evaluation report is good, the work-product reviewer would so inform the attorney and might assist in settlement, explanation of the report, or implementing its recommendations. It is when the report is sufficiently flawed that the work-product reviewer's role might change from advising the attorney of the strengths and weaknesses of a report to becoming a testifying expert regarding those weaknesses (and on cross-examination, presumably also those strengths).

Non-Testifying Consultants

In terms of non-testifying consulting roles, from Court's perspective, the Court may never know of the existence of the consultant unless the consultant actually comes to court to assist the attorney. If the consultant does come to court, the FMHP should be mindful of the judge's perception of such a consultant if the assistance occurs after FMHP has served in a testifying capacity (switching hats?). The FMHP and attorney might also consider the judge's perception even if the consultant has not testified, if the consultant has any communication with the parent-litigant in front of the judge (such as at counsel table).

When the FMHP works directly with the parent-litigant, as at least one of the articles in this issue discusses, there are certain dangers to consider, especially if there is a chance that the matter will ever be litigated. If a FMHP becomes part of a "team" to assist one parent in functioning post-separation, this becomes more like therapy, whether it is called "coaching," "parent education" or "consultation." Few would find fault in a parent who sincerely sought to better his or her parenting skills post-separation. (Some have expressed concern about doing even that if a child custody evaluation is pending. I respectfully decline to share that concern, however, because evaluations are, at best, a "snapshot in time" of a family in transition. The length of time from an order for an evaluation to the post-evaluation hearing can be extremely long, and children have to be parented in-between. If children can be parented well because the parents learn better ways to parent, I have little concern as to whether this skews data for the Court.)

If a FMHP works directly with a parent-litigant, there is a continuum of participation to be considered from the clearly ethical (explaining the stages of the evaluation, its duration and the component parts of a report) to the clearly unethical (providing the parent-litigant responses to psychometric tests in advance to appear more positive to the evaluator than truthful responses would yield). Both the legal and mental health fields have proscriptions from assisting others in perpetrating a fraud on the Court.

None of the authors argue that the FMHP consultant should attempt to perpetrate a fraud on the Court by portraying a parent falsely or providing false information to the Court; however, there is not unanimity as to what it means to "portray a parent falsely." Certainly, if a parent has spanked a child in the past it would be inappropriate for a MHP or an attorney to instruct the parent to falsely state, to an evaluator or a Court, that the parent had not done so. If the parent, in the course of separation and divorce, becomes educated about child-rearing and child development and, as a result of that information, determines to no longer ever spank the child, would it be false for the parent to tell an evaluator or a Court as much?

There is some tension between those who describe "consultation" exclusively as a litigation role for a FMHP and those who consider "consultation" as something which can go beyond to actually assist parents directly—in some cases, helping them avoid litigation entirely, which many would describe as a net gain for most families. Judges are encouraged to avoid making custody decisions where it is possible for parents to make them. For this reason judges appreciate mental health practitioners who assist parents to work out a parenting plan that is best for their families. This is, however, more often in a therapeutic role or a mediative role.

Mental health professionals who prepare attorneys by helping them understand psycho-legal issues—and help craft questions that will make testimony clearer for the judge–also do a service for the court (as well as for the attorneys and parent-litigants). Those who "polish" the parent-litigant by reducing the parent-litigant's anxiety about the process and help the parent-litigant present his or her best self, may also be assisting the process. Those who "sandpaper" the parent-litigant by trying to reshape the parent-litigant into something he or she is not often do more harm than good to that parent-litigant. After all, when you use sandpaper to reshape something, inevitably you end up exposing what is underneath, for good or bad.

NOTE

1. Rashomon is the 1950 crime mystery film directed by Akira Kurasawa in which four witnesses to a rape report the events from their own perspectives, and far differently from each other. The phenomenon of subjective vantage point observation has come to be known as the Rashomon Effect.

Index

www.routledge.com/ 9780415500548

Related titles from Routledge

Mothers, Infants and Young Children of September 11, 2001

A Primary Prevention Project

Edited by Beatrice Beebe, Phyllis Cohen, K. Mark Sossin and Sara Markese

The group of papers presented in this volume represents ten years of involvement of a group of eight core therapists, working originally with approximately forty families who suffered the loss of husbands and fathers on September 11, 2001. The project focuses on the families of women who were pregnant and widowed in the disaster, or of women who were widowed with an infant born in the previous year.

In 2011, marking the 10th anniversary of the World Trade Center tragedy, the Project continues to provide services without cost for these mothers who lost their husbands, for their infants who are now approximately ten years old, and for the siblings of these children.

This book was originally published as a special issue of the *Journal of Infant, Child and Adolescent Psychotherapy.*

February 2012: 246 x 174: 272pp
Hb: 978-0-415-50054-8
Pb: 978-0-415-50779-0
Hb: £80 / $125 Pb: £24.99 / $39.95

For more information and to order a copy visit
www.routledge.com/9780415500548

Available from all good bookshops

www.routledge.com/9780415570992

Related titles from Routledge

Mental Health Ethics
The Human Context
Edited by Phil Barker

All human behaviour is, ultimately, a moral undertaking, in which each situation must be considered on its own merits. As a result ethical conduct is complex. Despite the proliferation of Codes of Conduct and other forms of professional guidance, there are no easy answers to most human problems. *Mental Health Ethics* encourages readers to heighten their awareness of the key ethical dilemmas found in mainstream contemporary mental health practice.

This text provides an overview of traditional and contemporary ethical perspectives and critically examines a range of ethical and moral challenges present in contemporary 'psychiatric-mental' health services

Offering detailed consideration of issues and dilemmas, *Mental Health Ethics* helps all mental health professionals keep people at the centre of the services they offer.

November 2010: 246 x 174: 378pp
Hb: 978-0-415-57099-2
Pb: 978-0-415-57100-5
eBook: 978-0-203-83905-8
Hb: £75 / $125 Pb: £23.99 / $41.95
eBook: £23.99 / $41.95

For more information and to order a copy visit
www.routledge.com/9780415570992

Available from all good bookshops

www.routledge.com/9780415574594

Related titles from Routledge

Emerging Topics on Father Attachment

Considerations in Theory, Context and Development

Edited by Lisa A. Newland, Harry S. Freeman and Diana D. Coyl

This book is the first of its kind to focus specifically on children's attachment to fathers, and explores the connections among fathering, family dynamics, and attachment relationships. It includes theoretical, methodological and research reports written by an interdisciplinary group of researchers from around the globe. The purpose of this book is to familiarize the reader with the conceptualization, measurement and provisions of the attachment bond between children and their fathers, from infancy through young adulthood and across diverse individual, family, community, and cultural systems.

This book was published as a special issue of *Early Child Development and Care*.

July 2010 (PB Direct January 2012): 246 x 174: 262pp
Hb: 978-0-415-57459-4
Pb: 978-0-415-50895-7
Hb: £80 / $125 PB Direct: £24.95 / $45.95

For more information and to order a copy visit
www.routledge.com/9780415574594

Available from all good bookshops

www.routledge.com/9780415582971

Related titles from Routledge

Professional Issues in Child and Youth Care Practice

Edited by Kiaras Gharabaghi

This book provides an overview of the core professional issues in the field of child and youth care practice. The author explores themes ranging from relationships and the exploration of Self to career building and field-specific approaches to management. The book is written from a pragmatic perspective, and serves both to advance current thinking in the field about professional issues as well as to provide the student of child and youth care practice and practitioners with practical and accessible approaches to developing a strong and sustainable professional identity. All of the themes in this book are explored within a context of ethical decision-making and practice approaches informed by a commitment to children's rights and empowerment.

This book was originally published as a special issue of *Child and Youth Services*.

June 2010 (PB Direct December 2011): 246 x 174: 236pp
Hb: 978-0-415-58297-1
Pb: 978-0-415-51822-2
Hb: £75 / $125 PB Direct: £24.95 / $45.95

For more information and to order a copy visit
www.routledge.com/9780415582971

Available from all good bookshops

www.routledge.com/9780789037619

Related titles from Routledge

Family Factors and the Educational Success of Children

Edited by William Jeynes

Family Factors and the Educational Success of Children addresses a wide range of family variables and a diverse array of family situations in order to understand the dynamics of the multifaceted relationship between family realities and educational outcomes of children. It provides research on building effective partnerships between parents and teaches the importance of parental style, parental involvement as a means of improving family life, the influence of family factors on children of color, and the role of religion in influencing family and educational dynamics.

This book was published as a double special issue of *Marriage and Family Review*.

August 2009: 234 x 156: 420pp
Hb: 978-0-7890-3761-9
Pb: 978-0-7890-3762-6
Hb: £80 / $130 Pb: £22.99 / $45.95

For more information and to order a copy visit
www.routledge.com/9780789037619

Available from all good bookshops

www.routledge.com/9780789037091

Related titles from Routledge

Social Work and Global Mental Health

Research and Practice Perspectives

Edited by Serge Dumont and Myreille St-Onge

This book presents respected experts, researchers, and clinicians providing the latest developments in social work knowledge and research. It discusses the latest in mental health research, information on violence, trauma and resilience, and social policies. Different mental health and social work approaches from around the world are examined in detail, including holistic, ethnopsychiatric, and interventions that place emphasis on recovery, empowerment, and social inclusion. This superb selection of presentations taken from the 4th International Conference on Social Work in Health and Mental Health held in Quebec, Canada in 2004 comprehensively examines the theme of how social work can contribute to the development of a world that values compassion and solidarity.

This book was originally published as a special issue of *Social Work in Mental Health*.

March 2009: 246 x 174: 306pp
Hb: 978-0-7890-3709-1
Pb: 978-0-7890-3710-7
Hb: £75 / $125 Pb: £25.99 / $49.95

For more information and to order a copy visit
www.routledge.com/9780789037091

Available from all good bookshops